Picky Nicky
The Nutrition Decision

Kids, You Are
What You Eat!

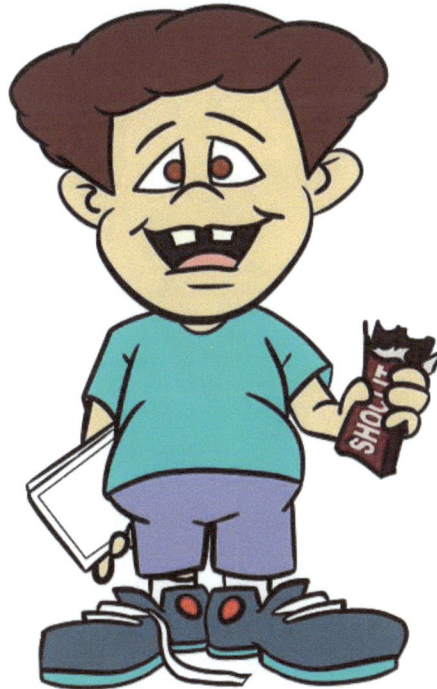

Written and Illustrated by
Christopher Silvestre
www.SilvestreArt.com

ISBN: 978-0692856741

Nicky is a boy who
dislikes healthy food.

Whenever Mom makes it,
he gets in a bad mood.

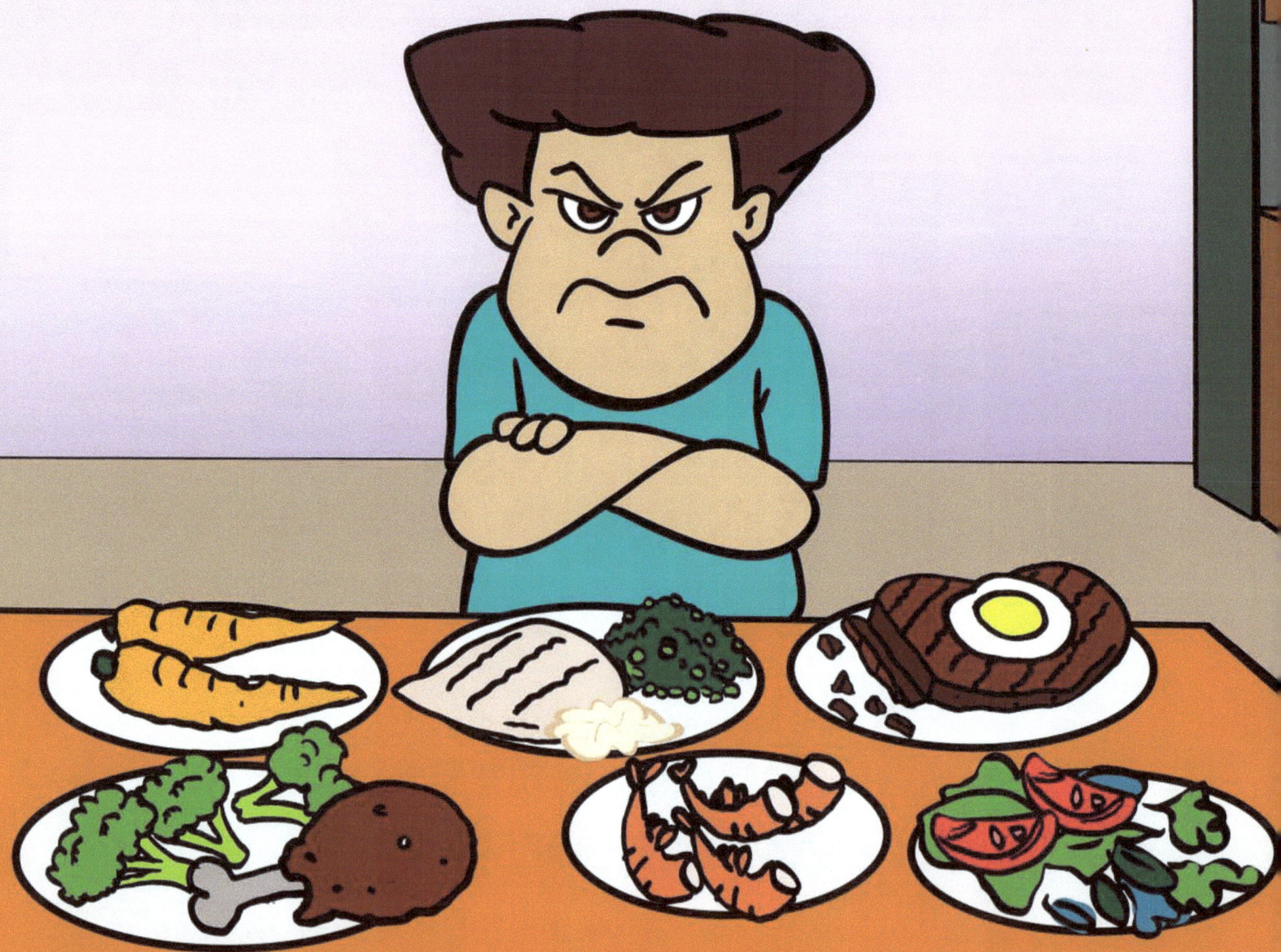

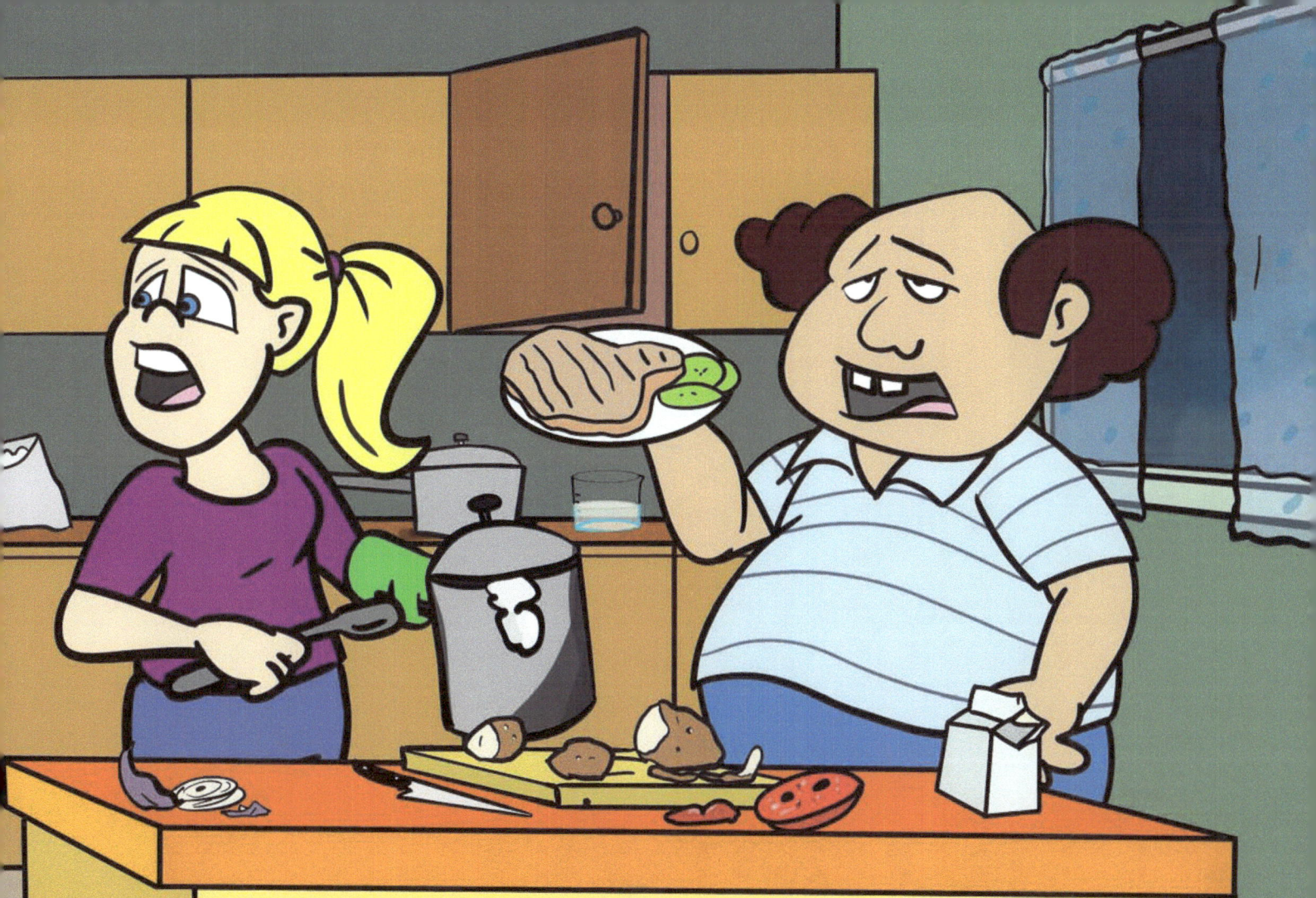

His parents, they pleaded,
"Nicky, try something new."
But Nicky is picky.
What else could they do?

He wouldn't eat chicken,
if they baked it or fried it.
He says he hates broccoli,
but he's never tried it.

No carrots. No fish.
No chili. No rice.
No turkey. No apples.
Don't even ask twice.

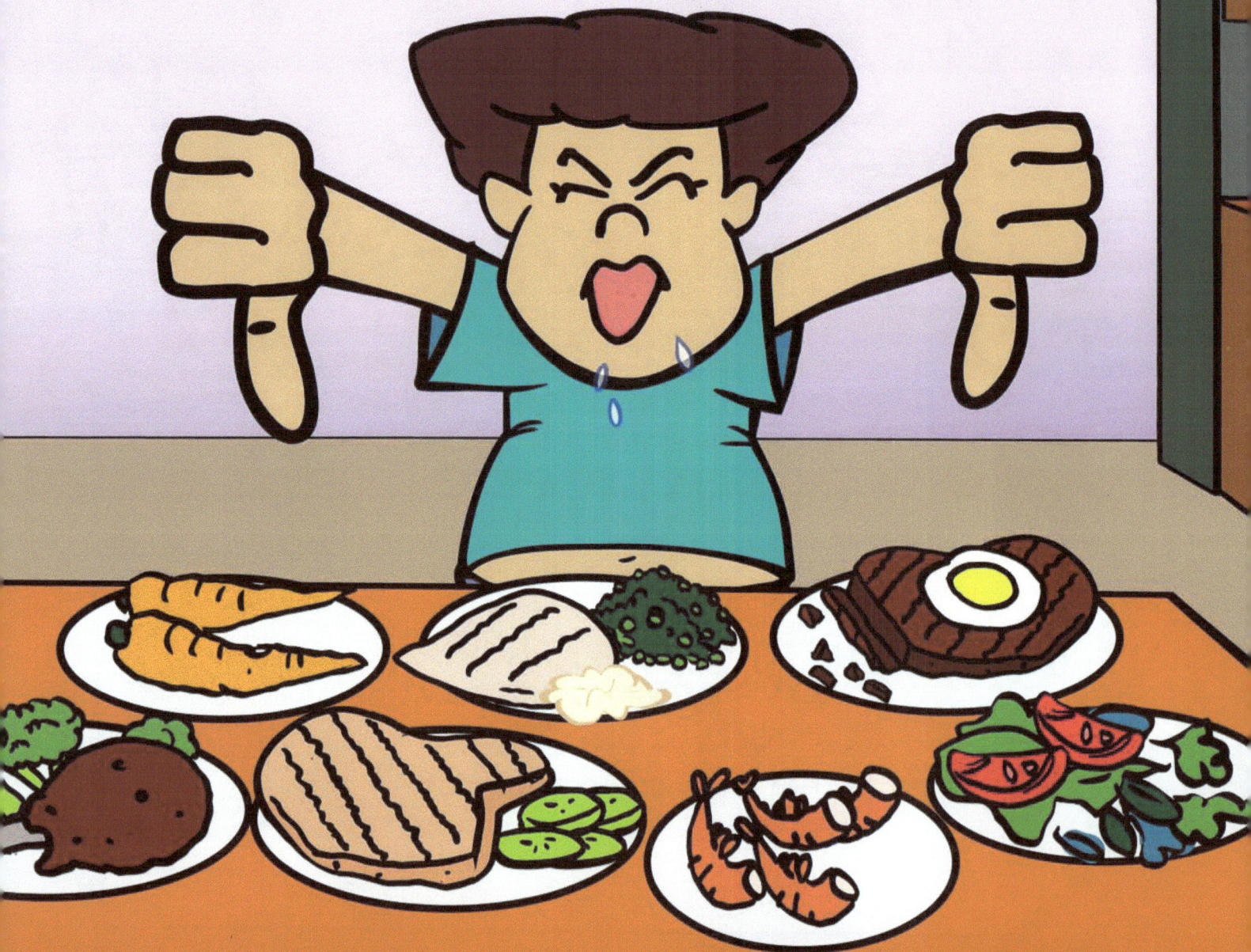

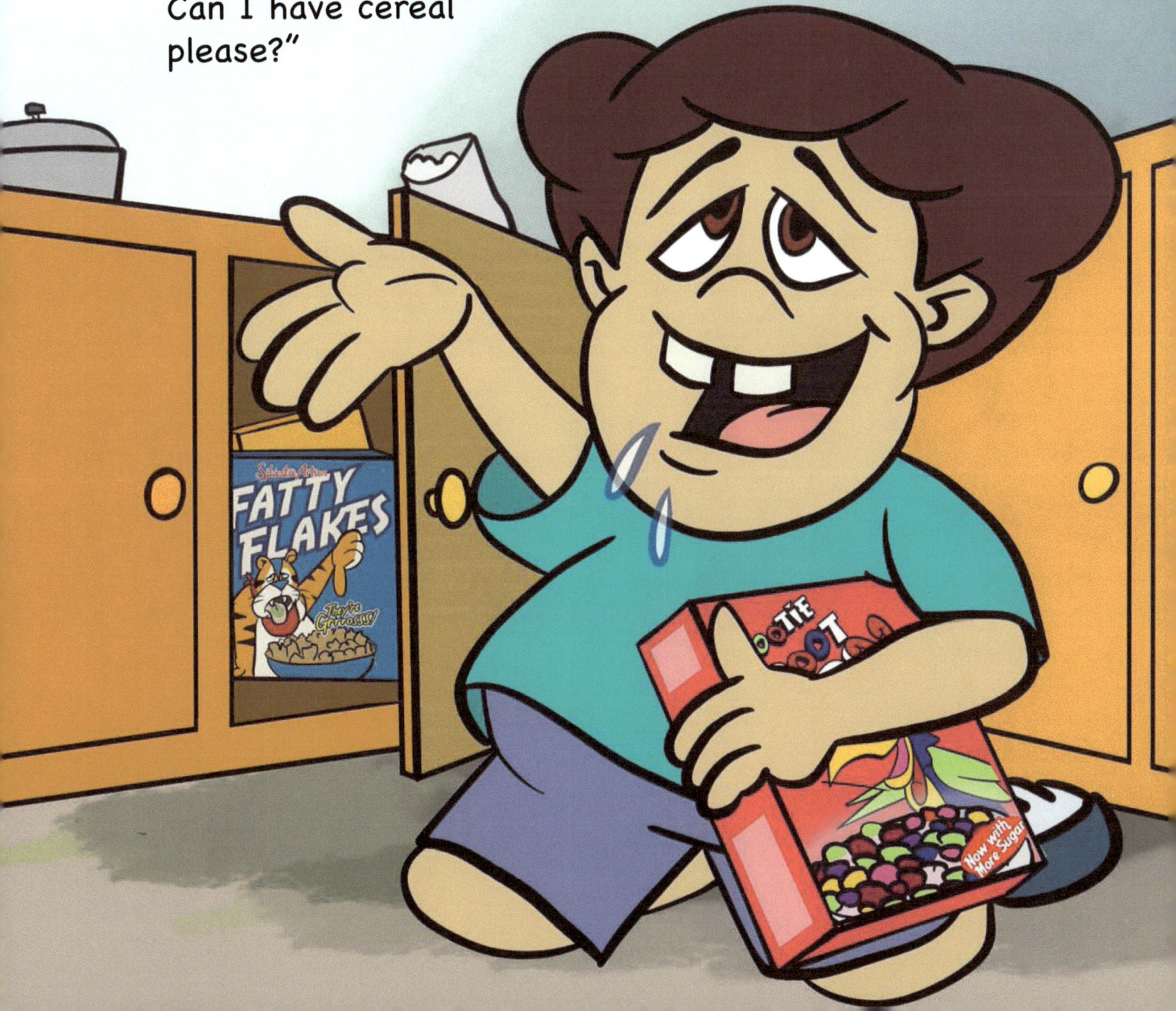

Nicky begged his parents
on his hands and his knees,
"I promise to be good.
Can I have cereal
please?"

So into his bowl
Frootie Froot Pops
were dumped.

Marshmallows
turned the milk pink.
The sugar started
to clump.

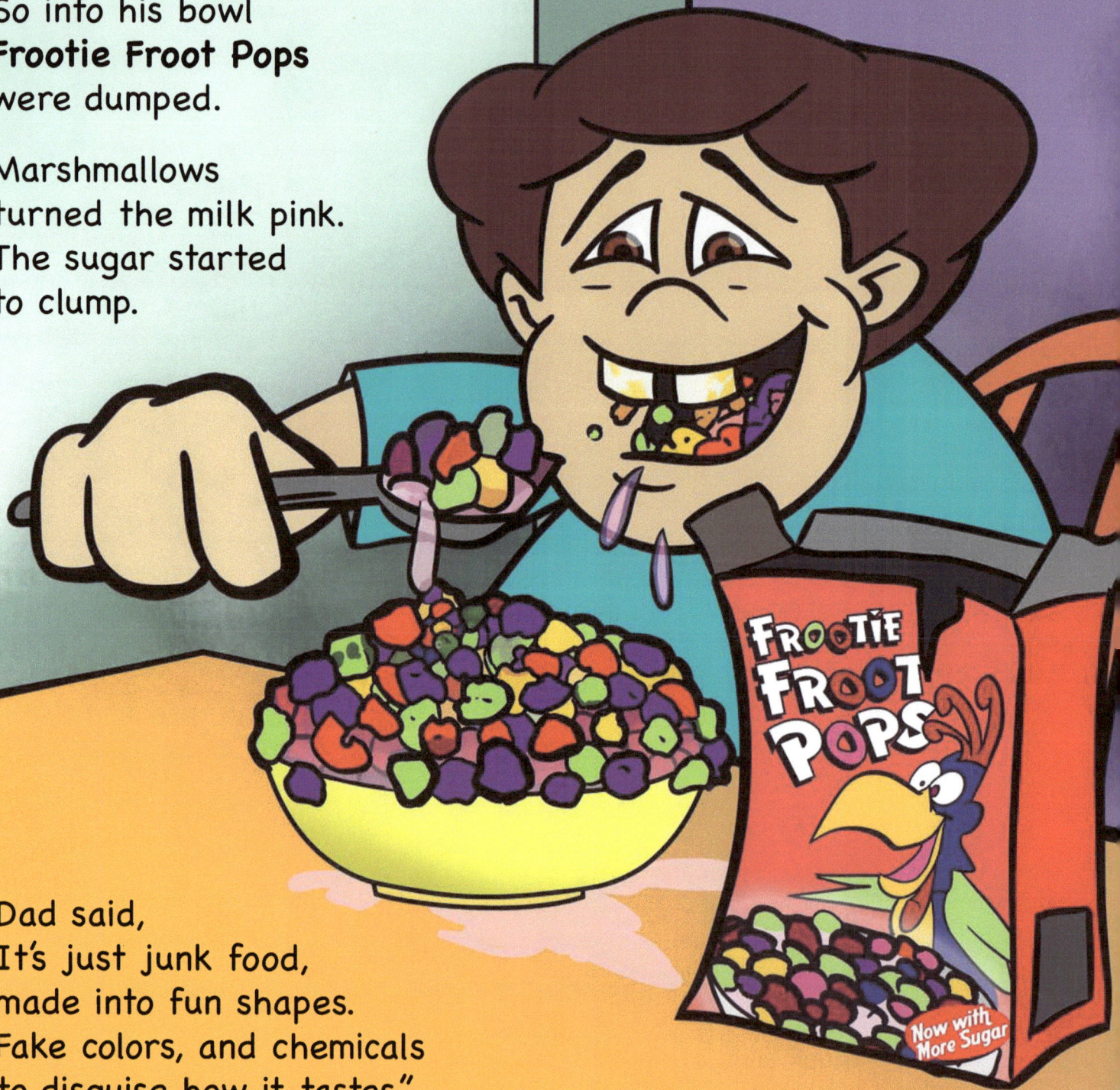

Dad said,
"It's just junk food,
made into fun shapes.
Fake colors, and chemicals
to disguise how it tastes."

FROOTIE
FROOT
POPS

Now with
More Sugar

Nicky just loved to eat
things that were squishy.

Like fruit snacks,
(**NOT** made from fruit)
and those little red fishies.

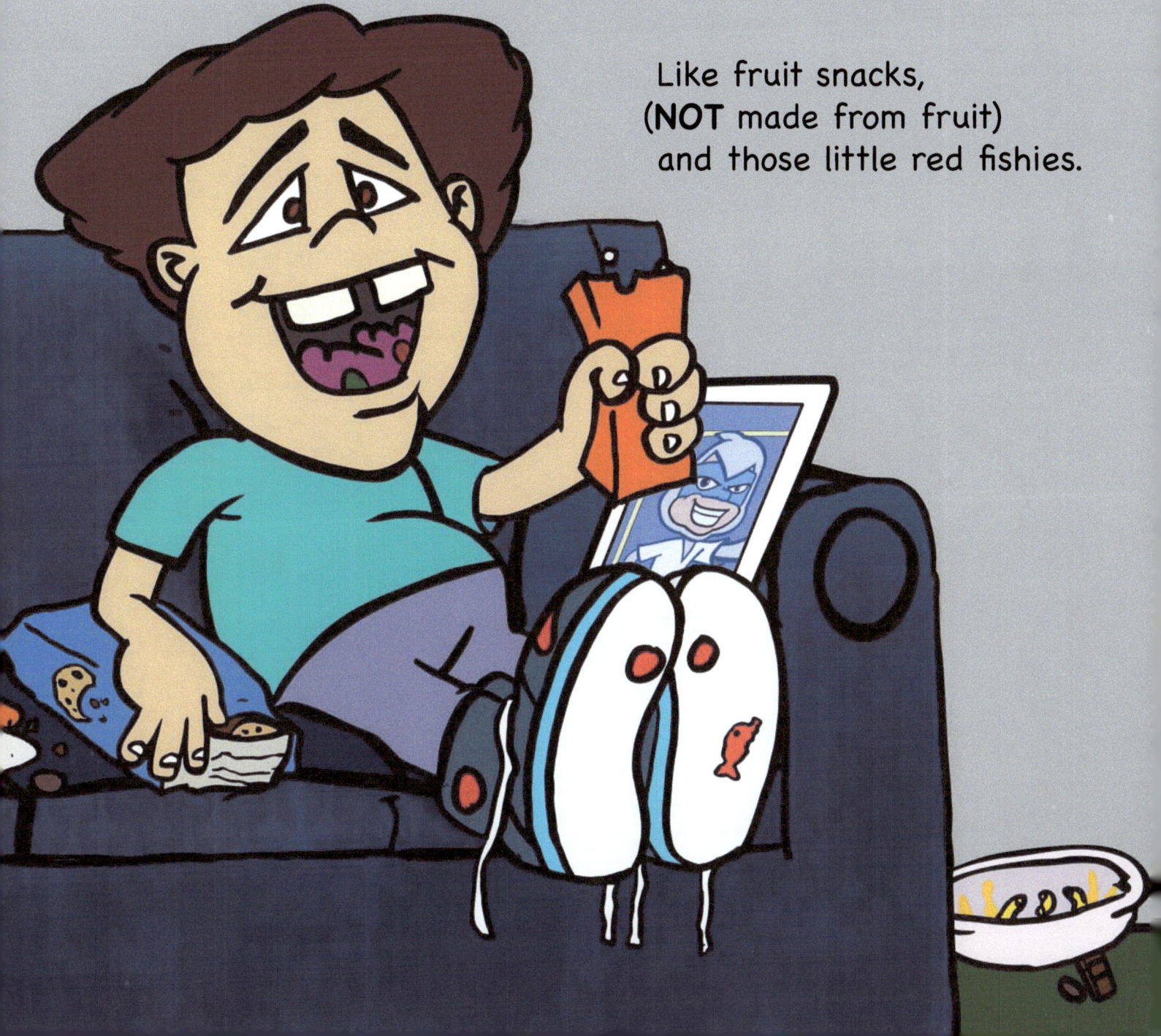

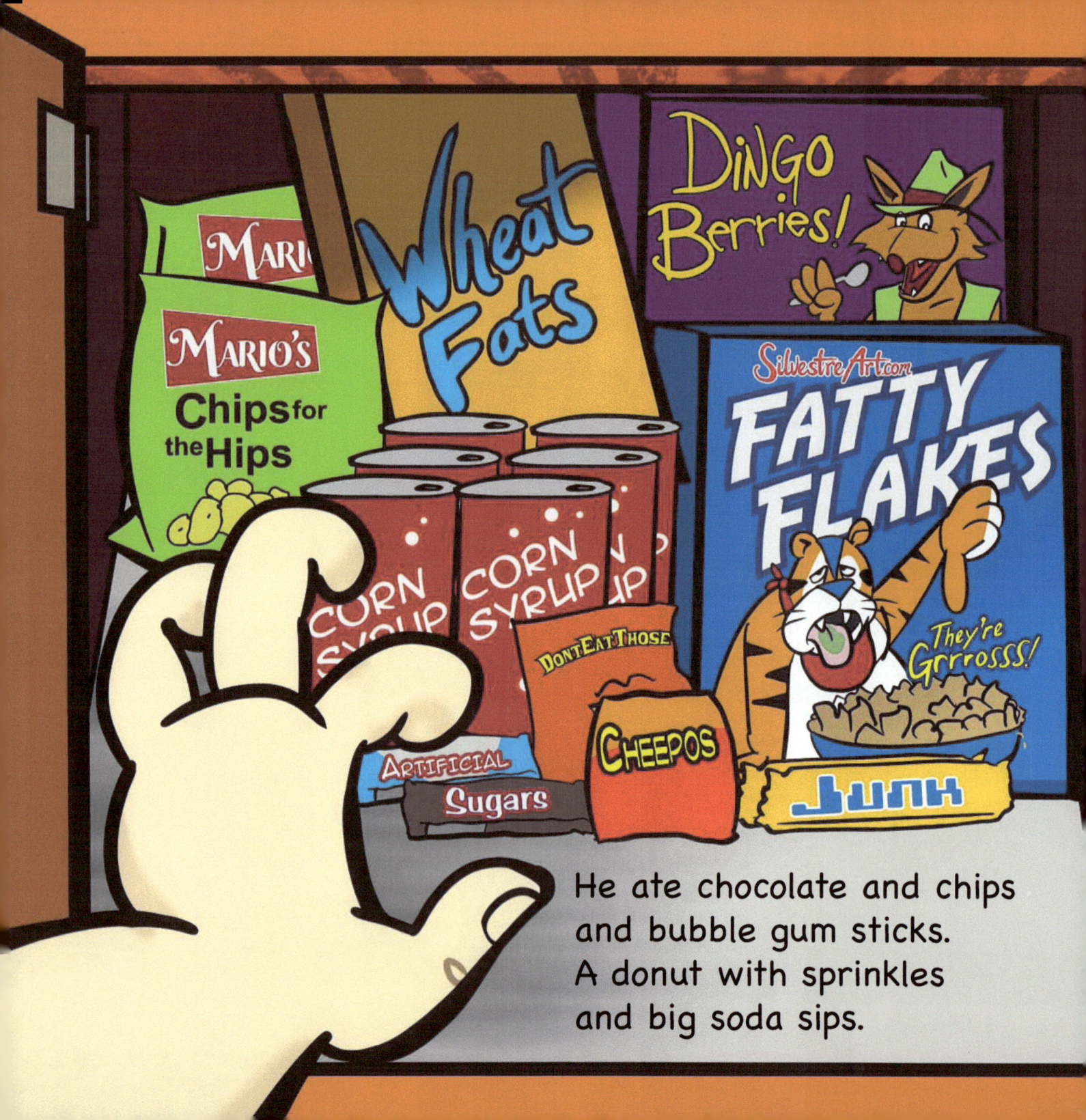

He ate chocolate and chips
and bubble gum sticks.
A donut with sprinkles
and big soda sips.

He ate 'til his tummy
was about to explode.
Then Nicky and his tablet
went into sleep mode.

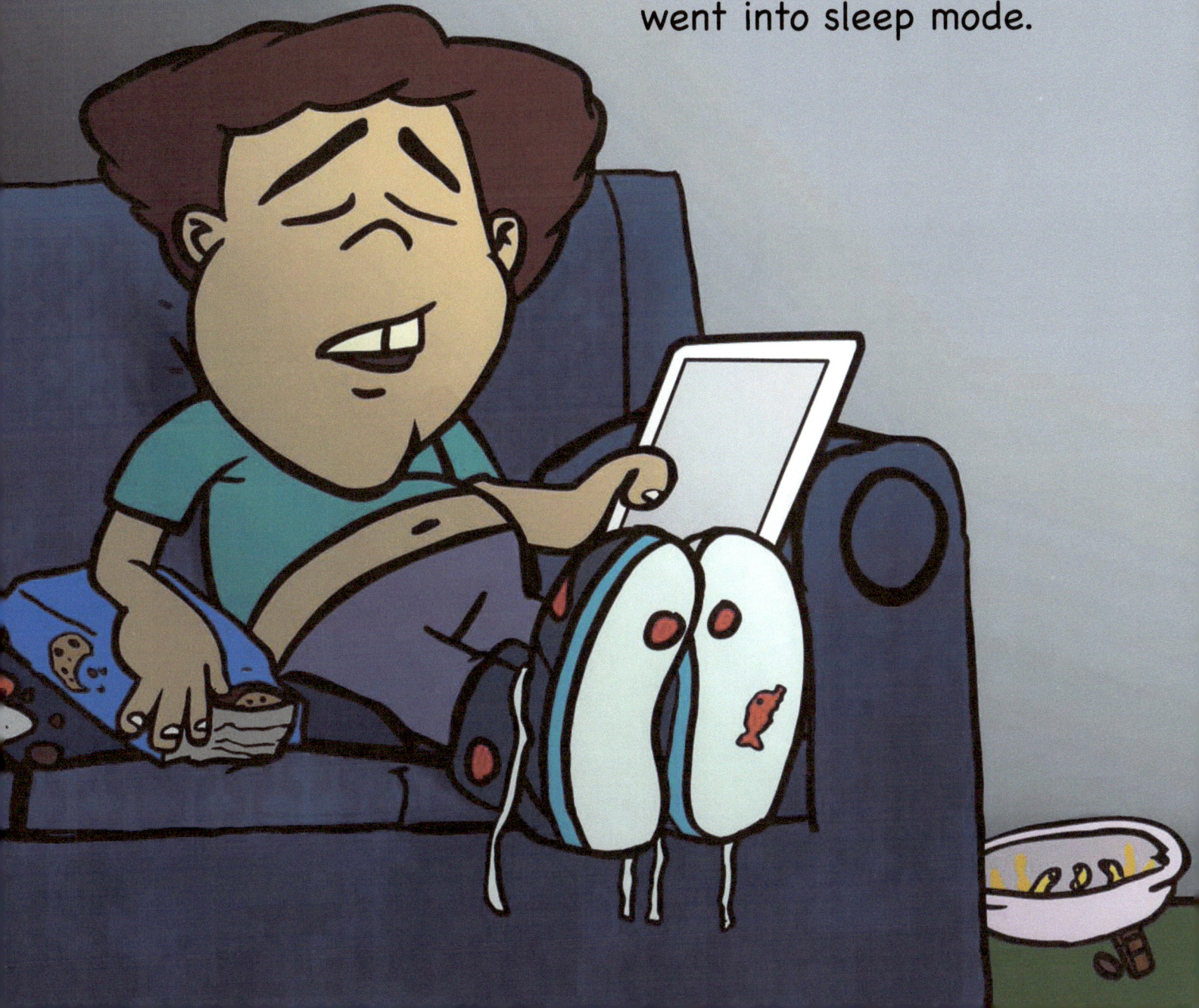

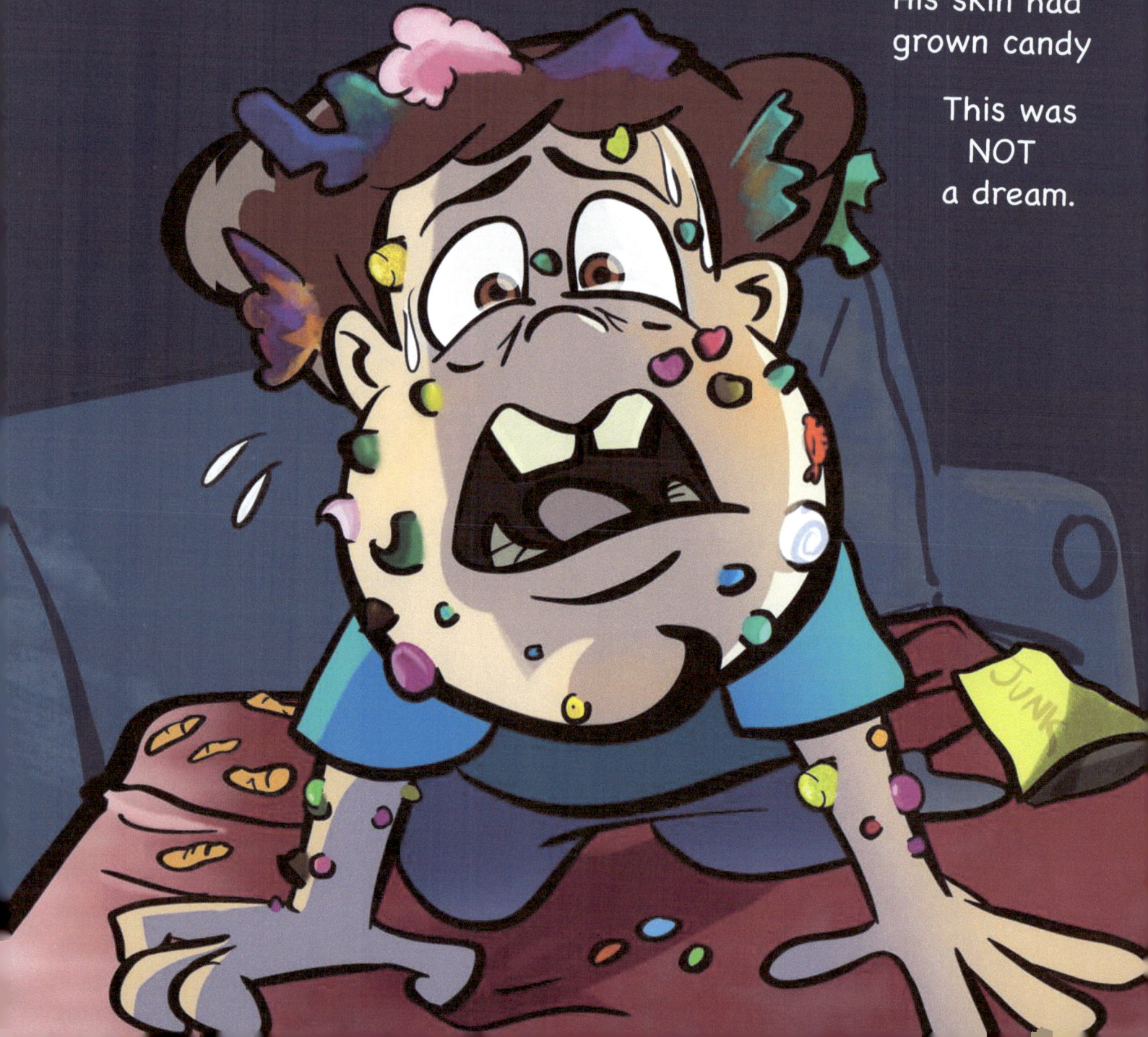

The next day Nicky woke up and he started to scream.

His skin had grown candy

This was NOT a dream.

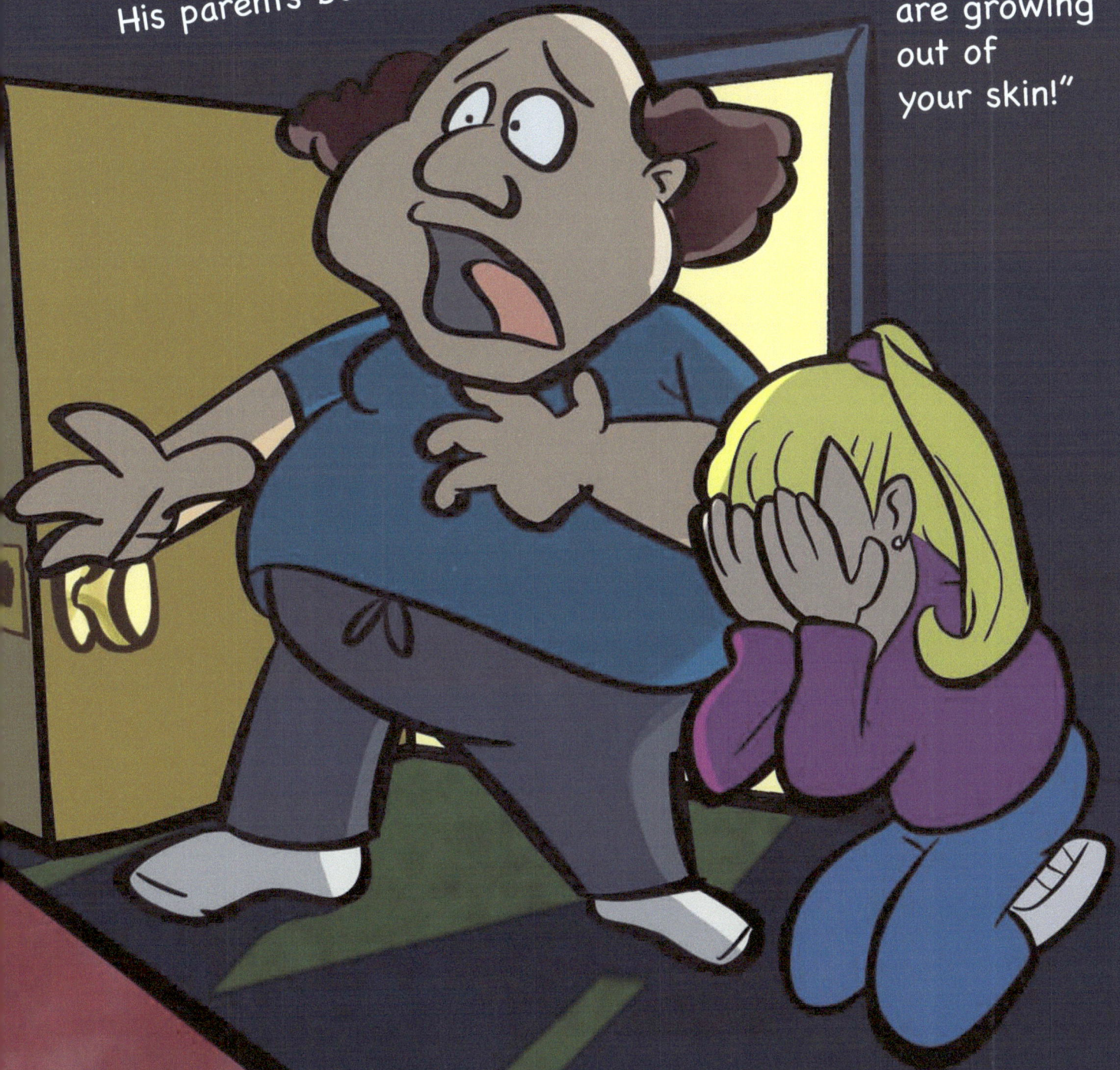

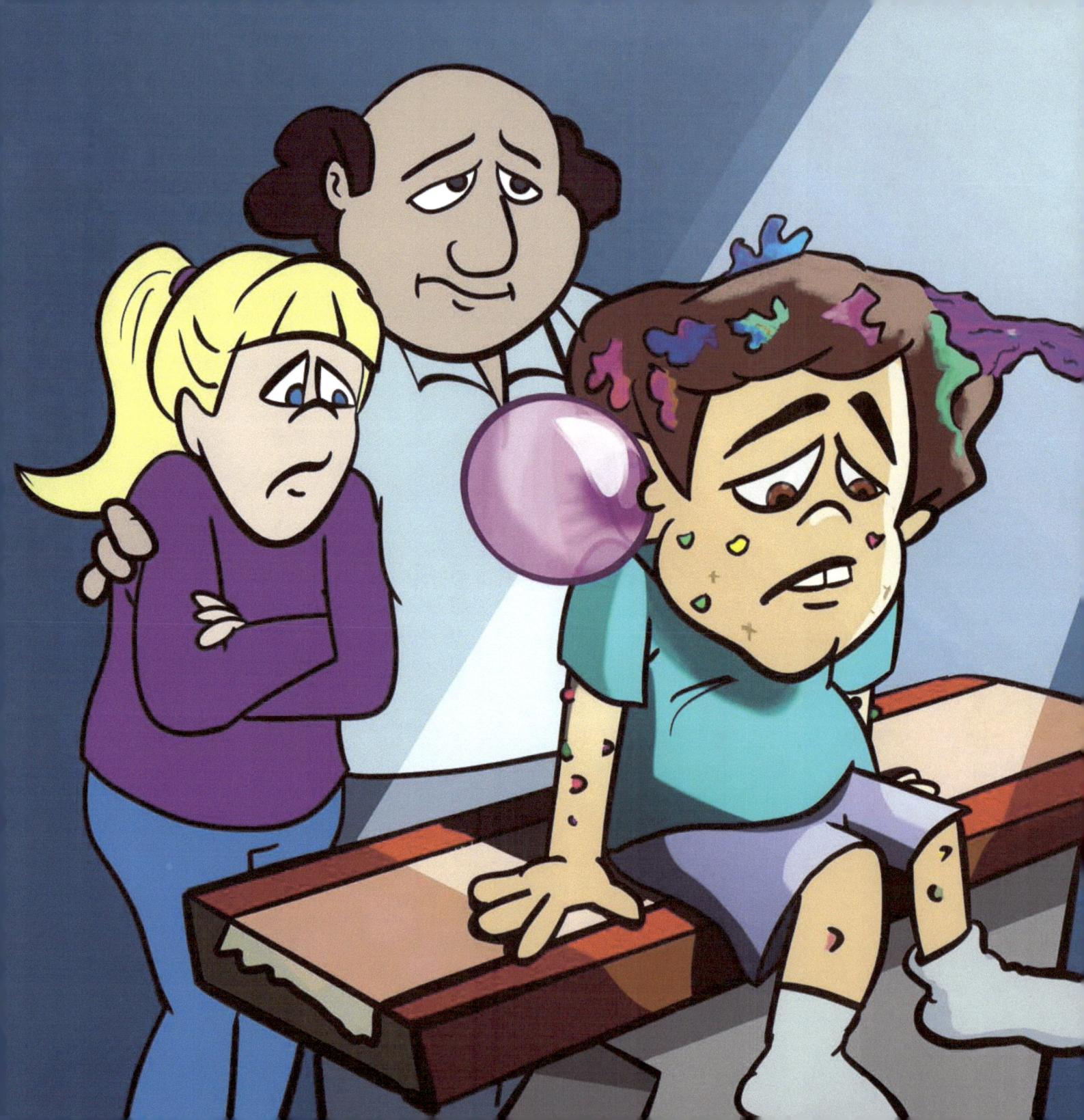

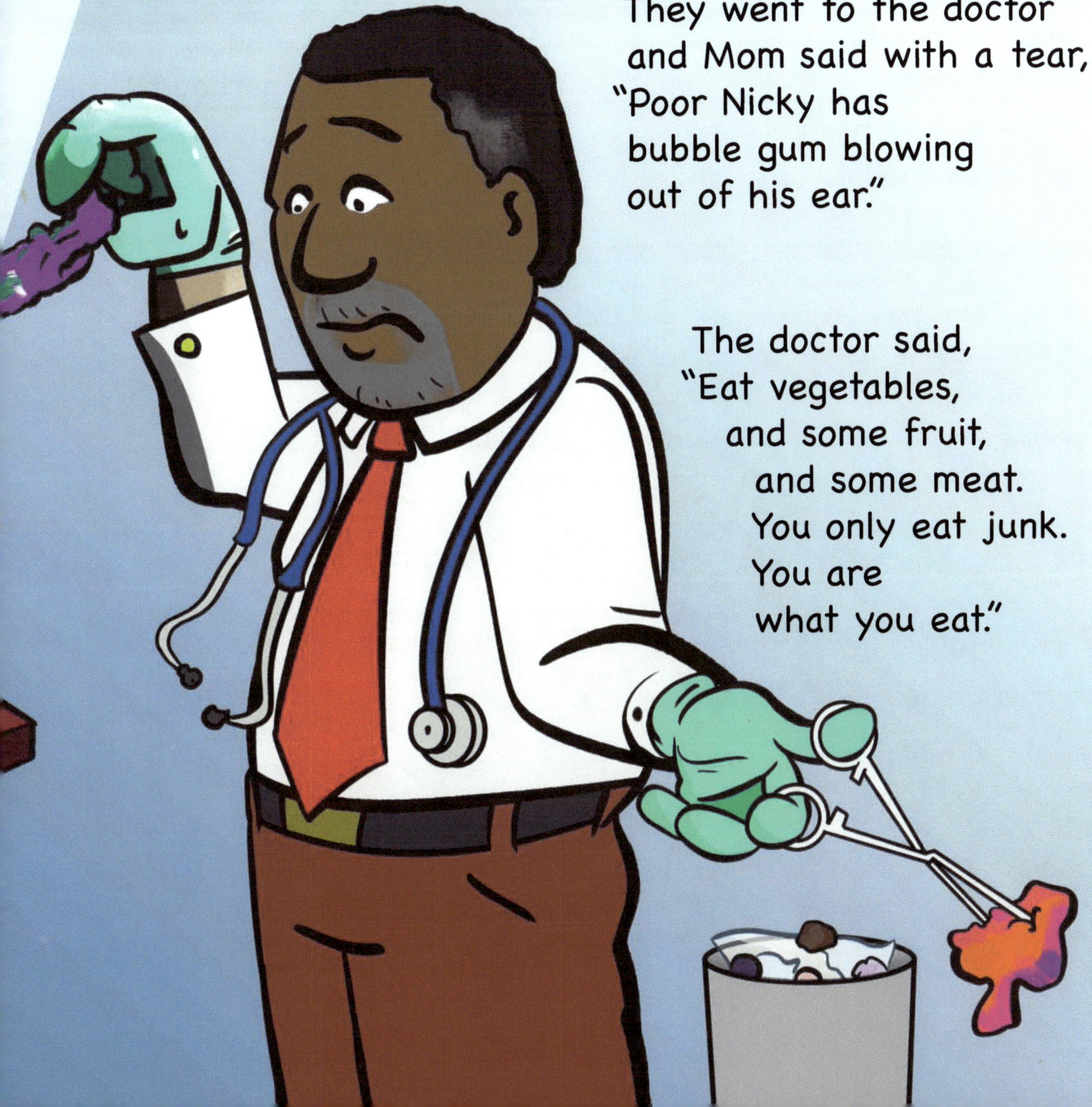

They went to the doctor and Mom said with a tear, "Poor Nicky has bubble gum blowing out of his ear."

The doctor said, "Eat vegetables, and some fruit, and some meat. You only eat junk. You are what you eat."

Nicky went shopping
with Mom and Dad
at the store.
They picked from a list
of fresh food to look for.

"We'll buy only good stuff
and learn one by one.
We'll cut out the garbage
and make healthy food fun!"

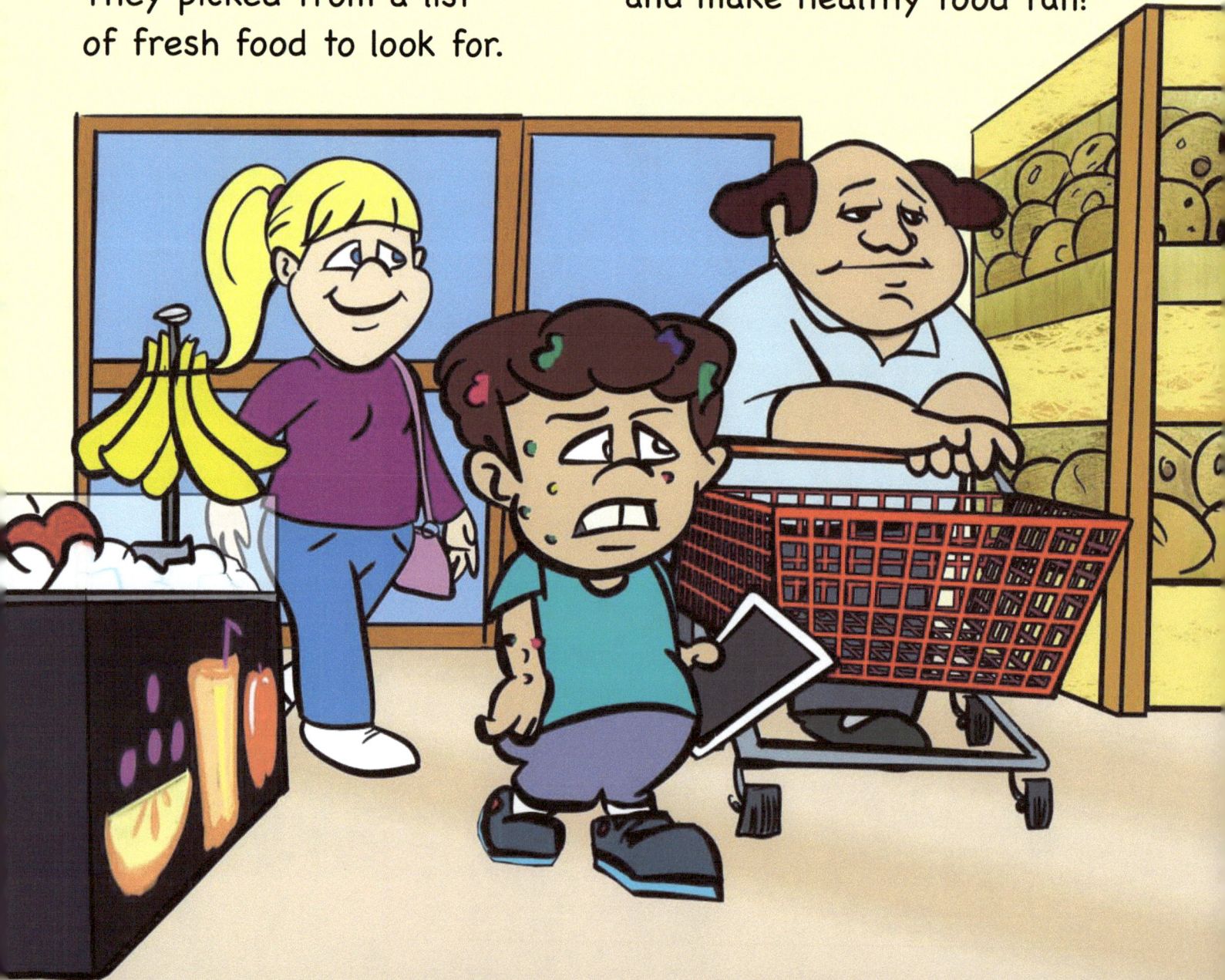

We eat
carbohydrates
to get up and go.
They give us the energy
to play and to throw.

Some wheat bread or fruit.
Some potatoes or rice.
A smoothie with blueberries
and bananas is nice.

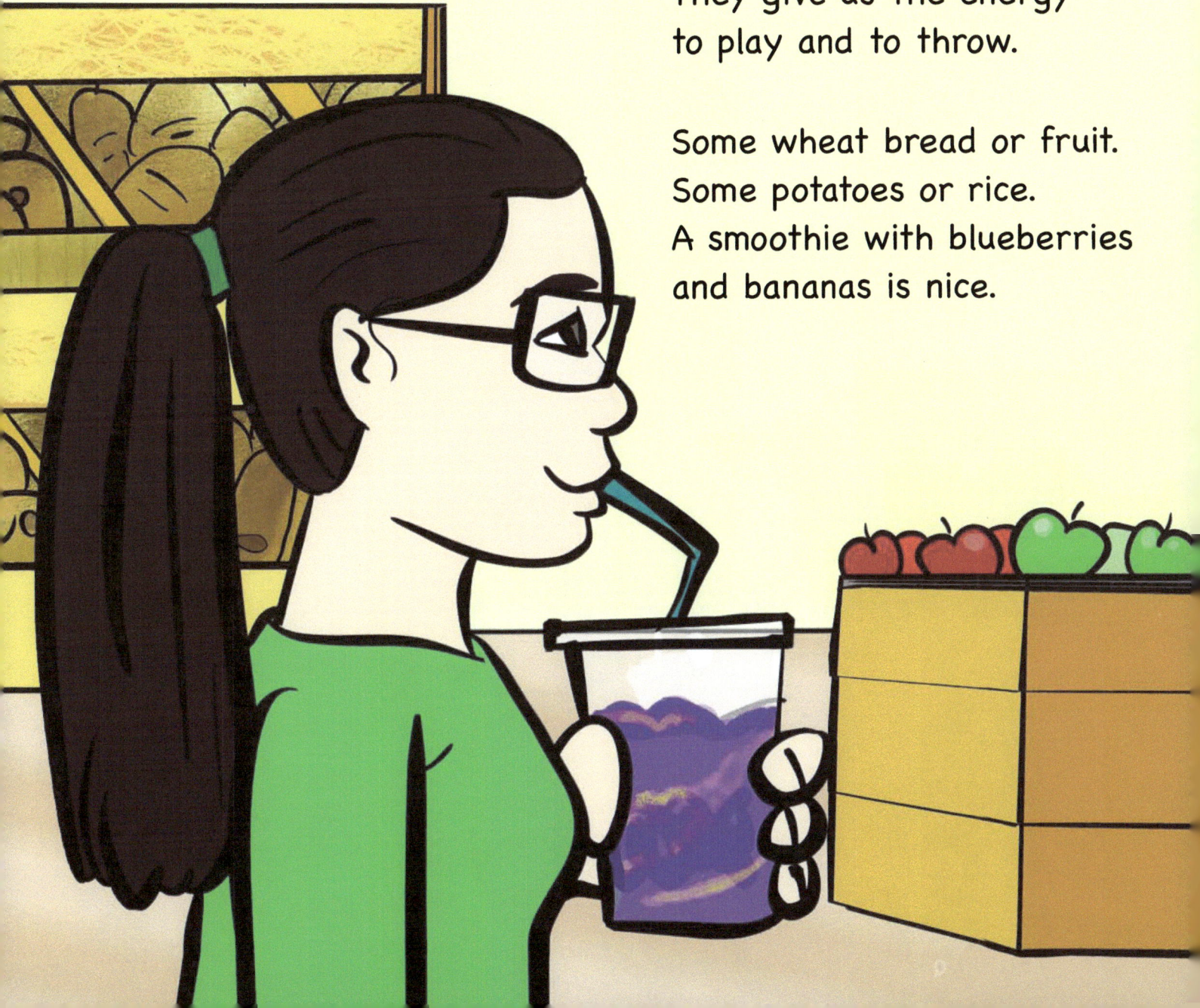

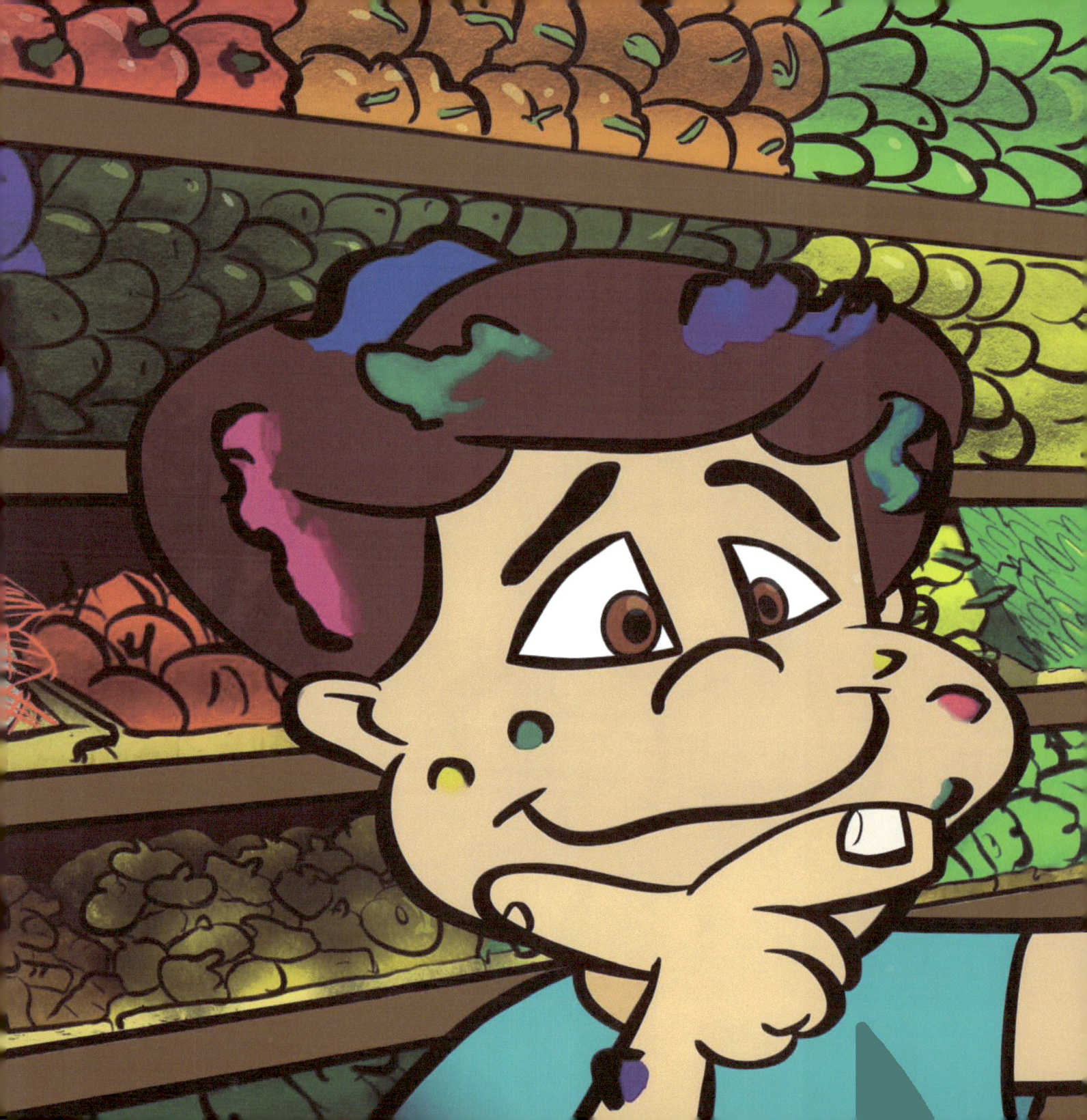

Vegetables can be orange, red, green, or brown.
These foods come from farms and grow out of the ground.

Vegetables are the best thing to put in your belly. They have vitamins and fiber to help keep us healthy.

We want to grow strong
and healthy and lean.
We build up our muscles
by eating **protein**.

Steak, fish, and chicken.
Milk, eggs, and nuts.
To build strong arms
and strong legs
and even strong butts.

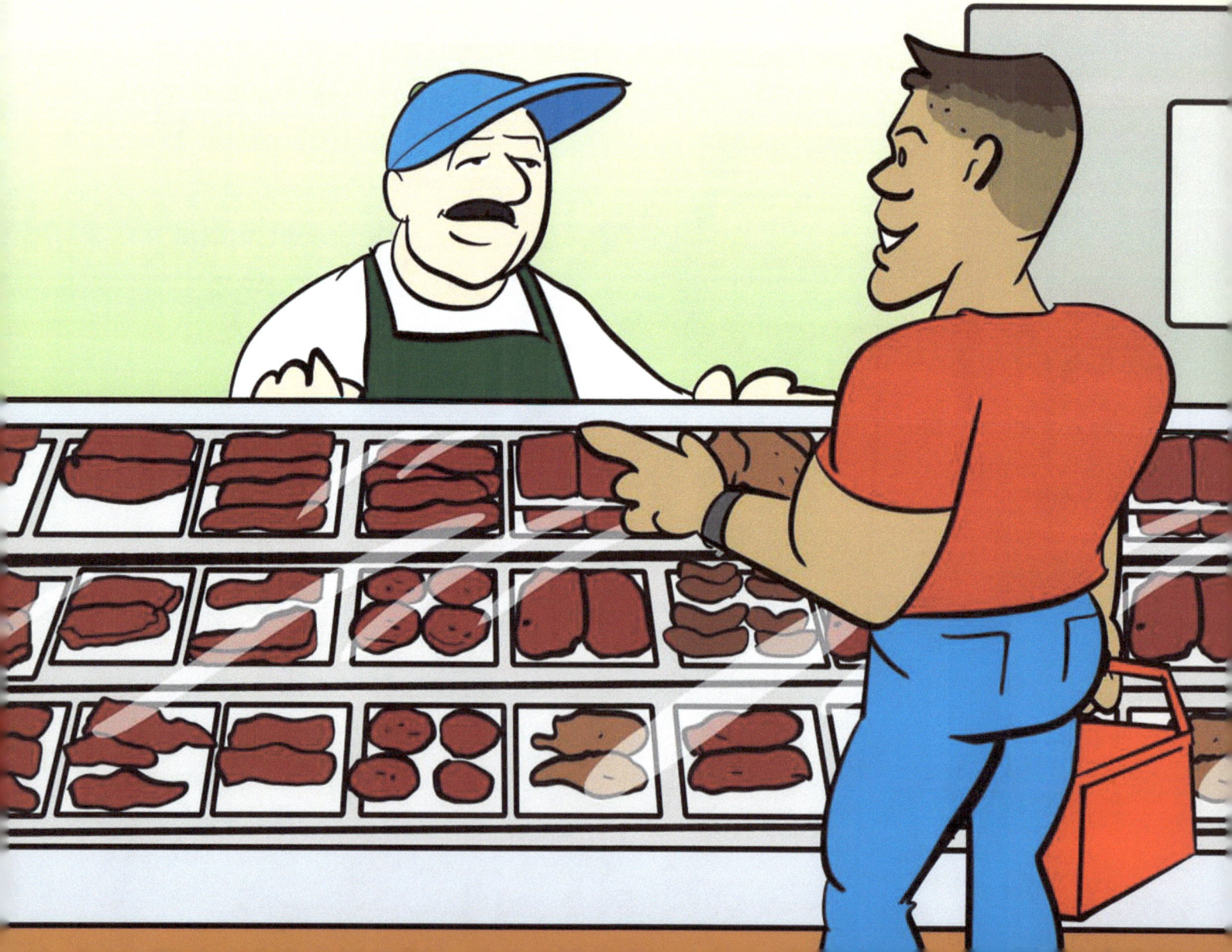

Nicky passed by the meats and cried, "They're disgusting!"

Then he licked up the drips from his chocolate chips busting.

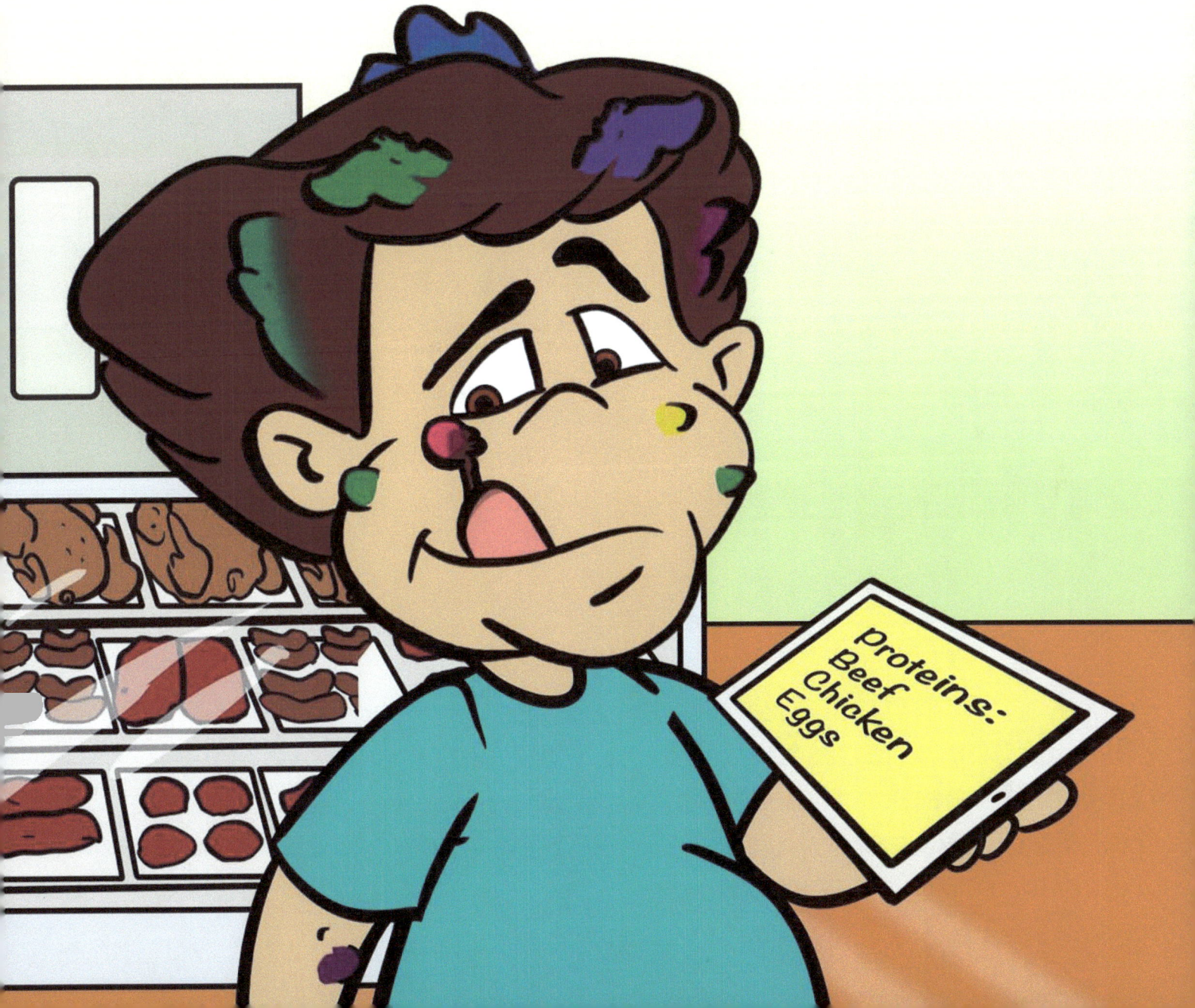

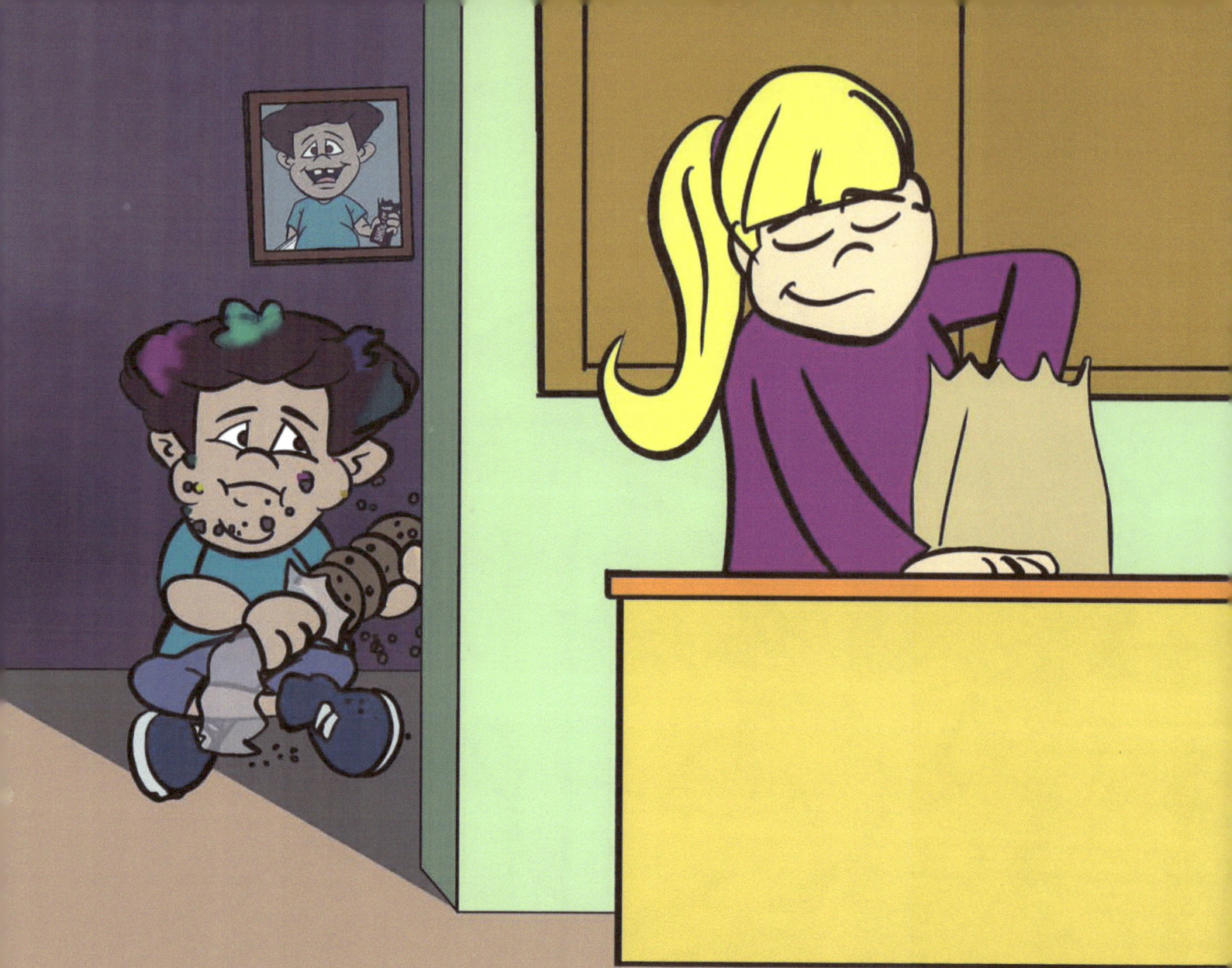

They got home with the food
to cook in the kitchen.
For dinner, Mom was making
some carrots and chicken.

But Nicky was hungry,
and Mom was still cooking.
So Nicky gobbled some cookies
when no one was looking.

Nicky plopped on the couch
and felt sluggish and drowsy.
Dinner was coming
but his belly felt lousy.

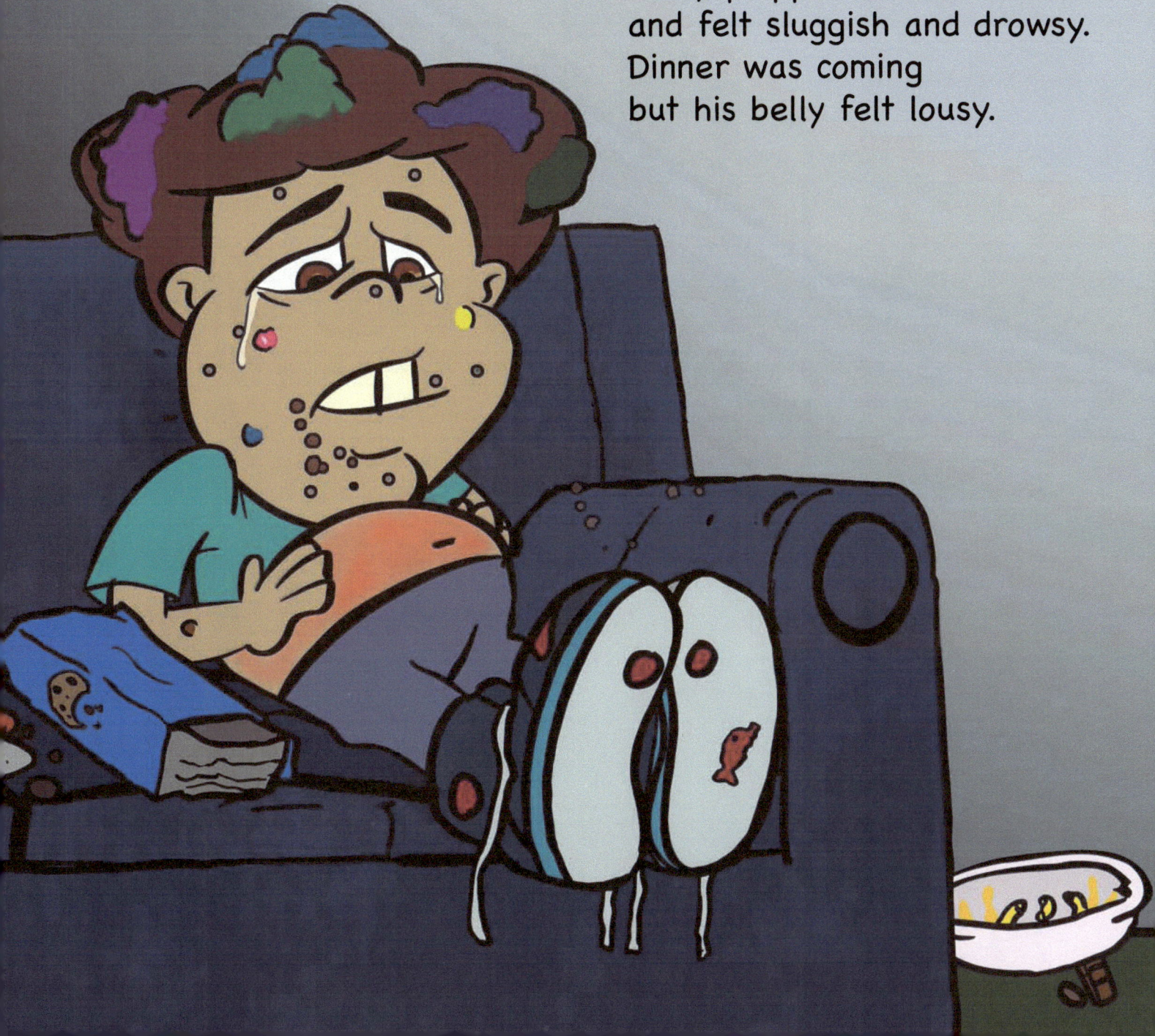

When they sat down for dinner Nicky took a small taste. He didn't like it and he spit it all over the place!

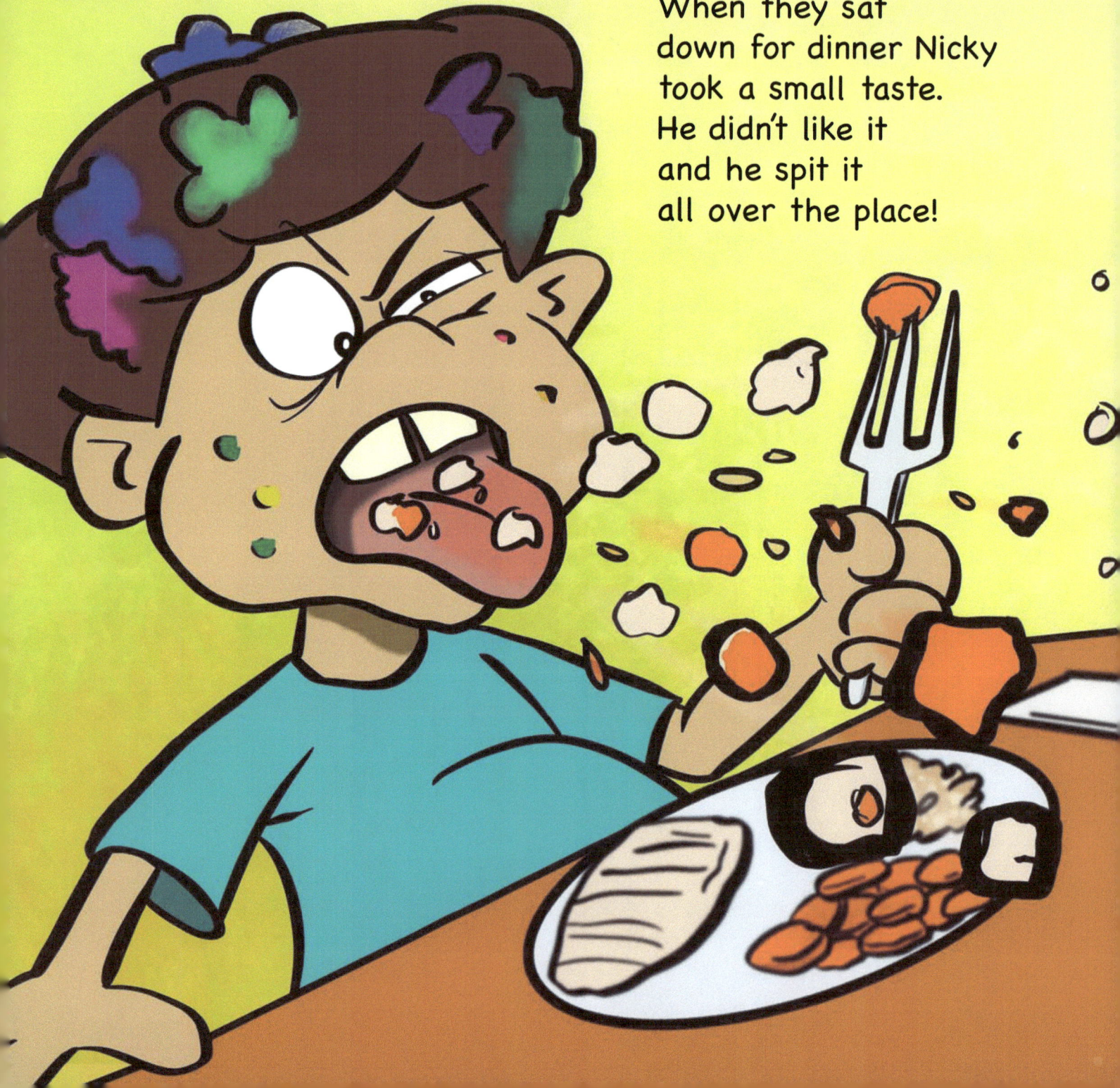

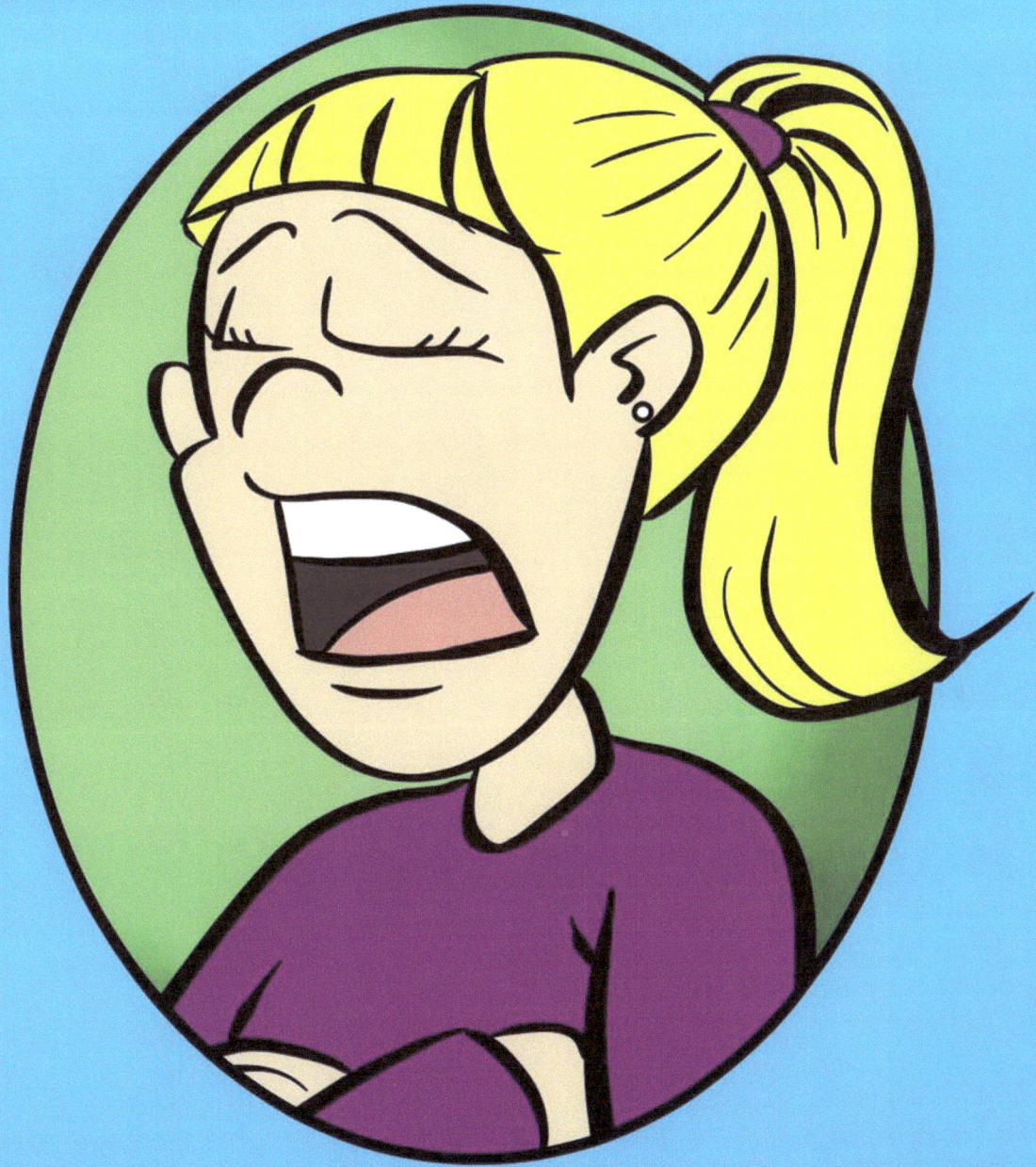

"Forget it!" Mom said,
"Nicky, make your own food."

"I'm not cooking for you
If you are gonna be rude."

Nicky went to make dinner
but was not feeling good.
Nicky wanted to eat healthy
if only he could.

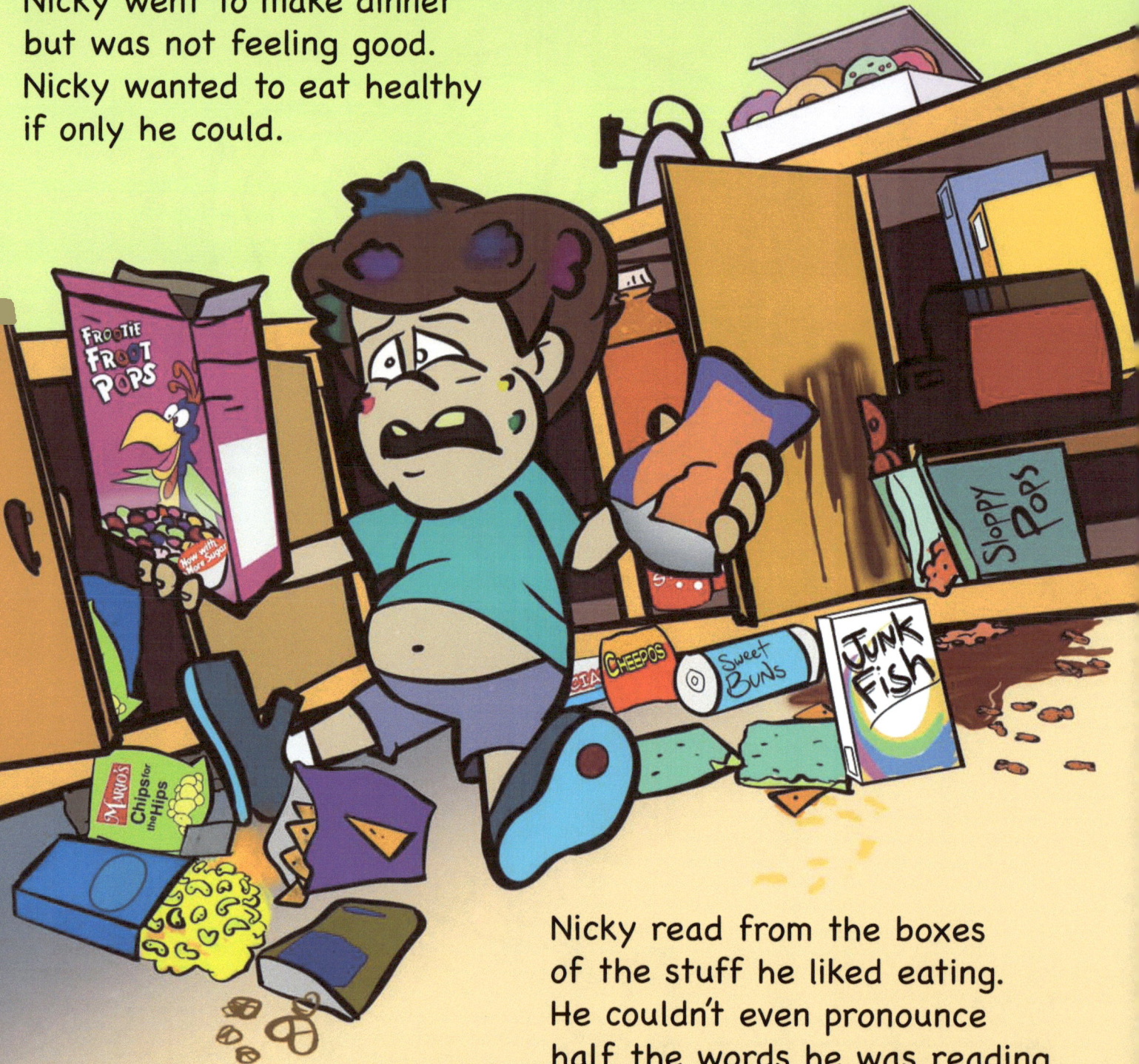

Nicky read from the boxes
of the stuff he liked eating.
He couldn't even pronounce
half the words he was reading.

There were cartoons on the boxes,
but that didn't matter,
because just eating junk food
makes kids bellies fatter.

His stomach still aching,
Nicky had no more doubt.
He took all of the junk food
and he threw it all out!

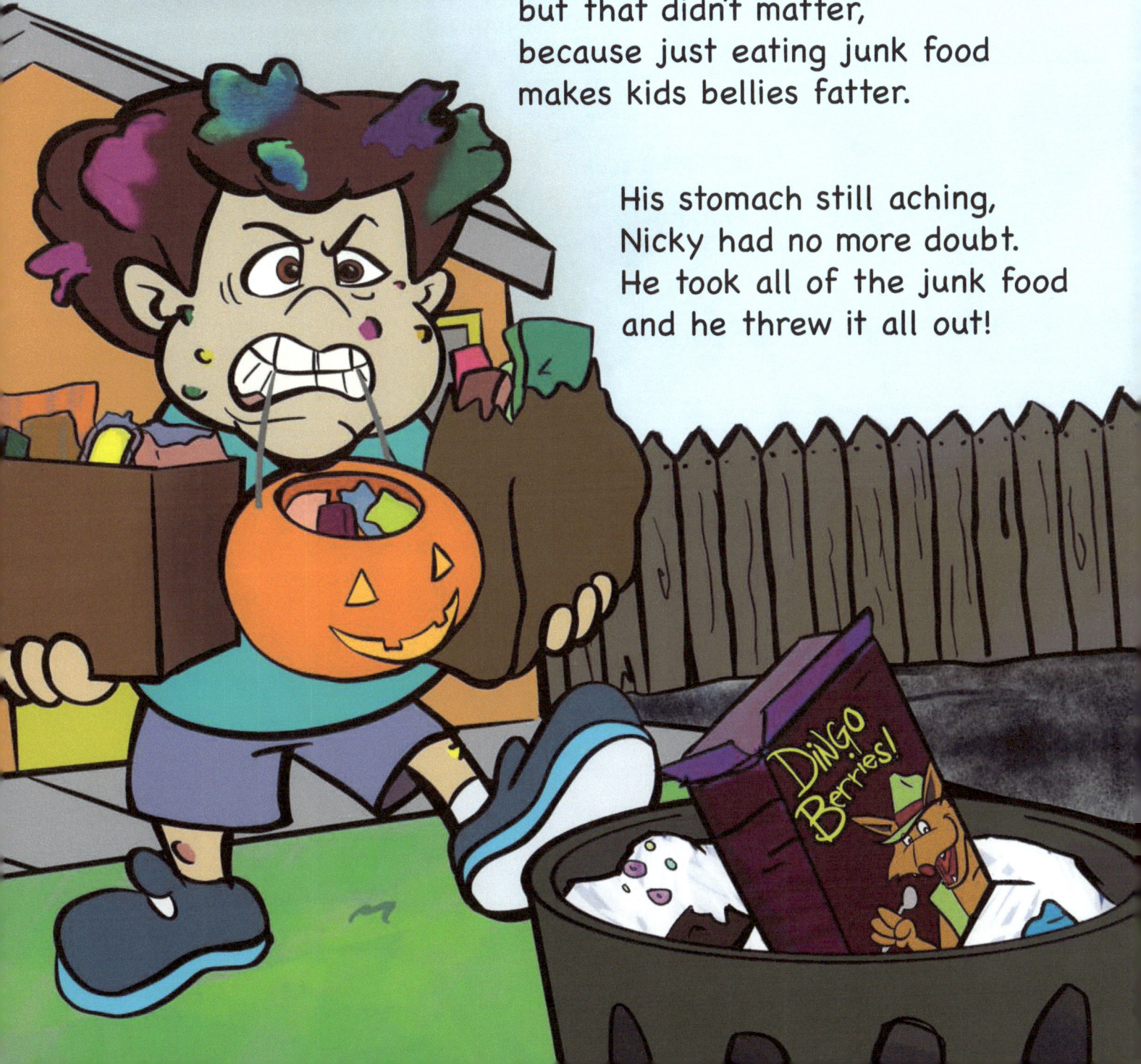

DiNGo Berries!

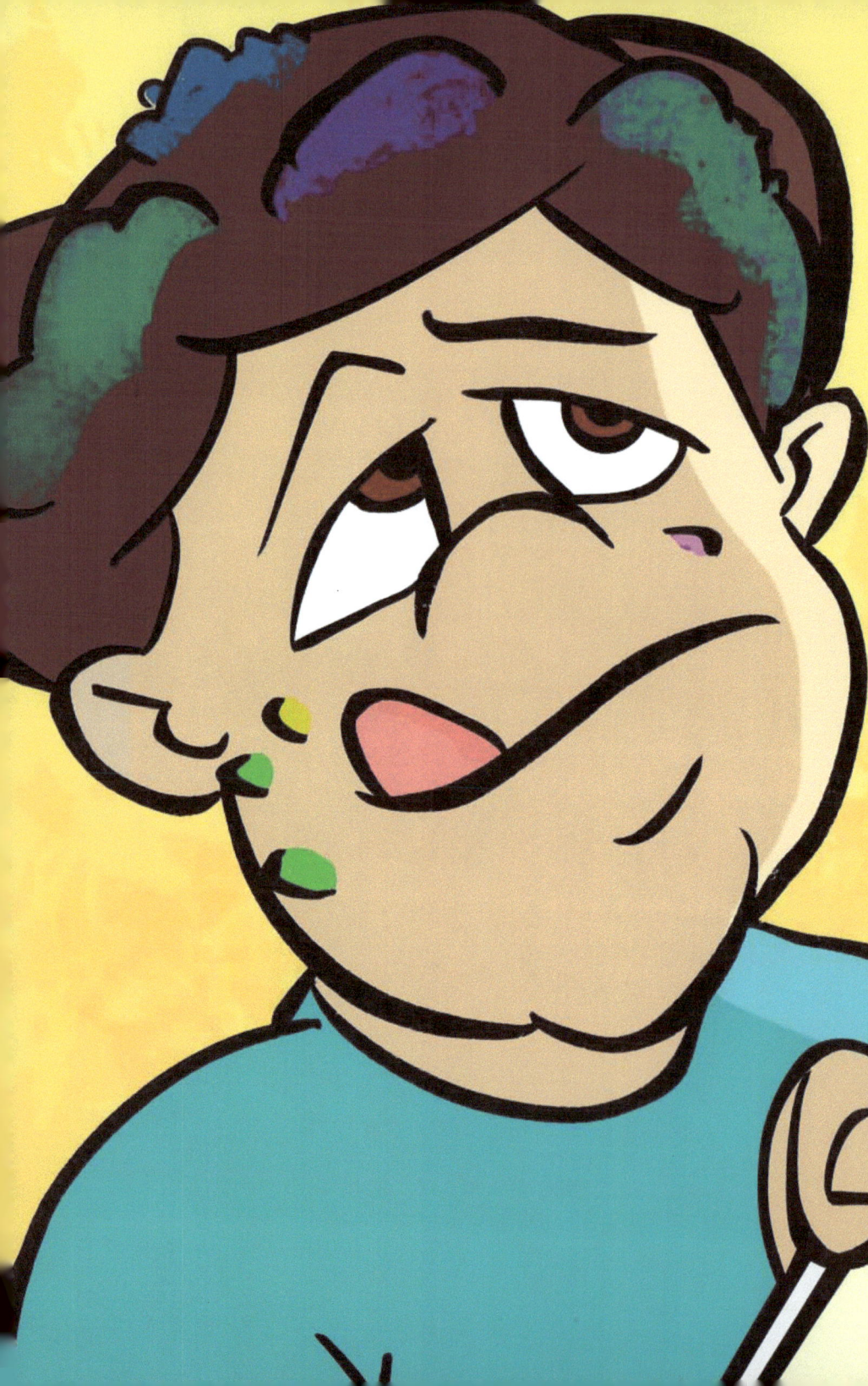

Nicky thought of some ways to make healthy food yummy.

So that he could start putting good things in his tummy.

- Make it
- Mix it
- Play with it

He pealed bananas for smoothies.
He washed veggies for stew.
It's fun to help **MAKE** things
you are planning to chew.

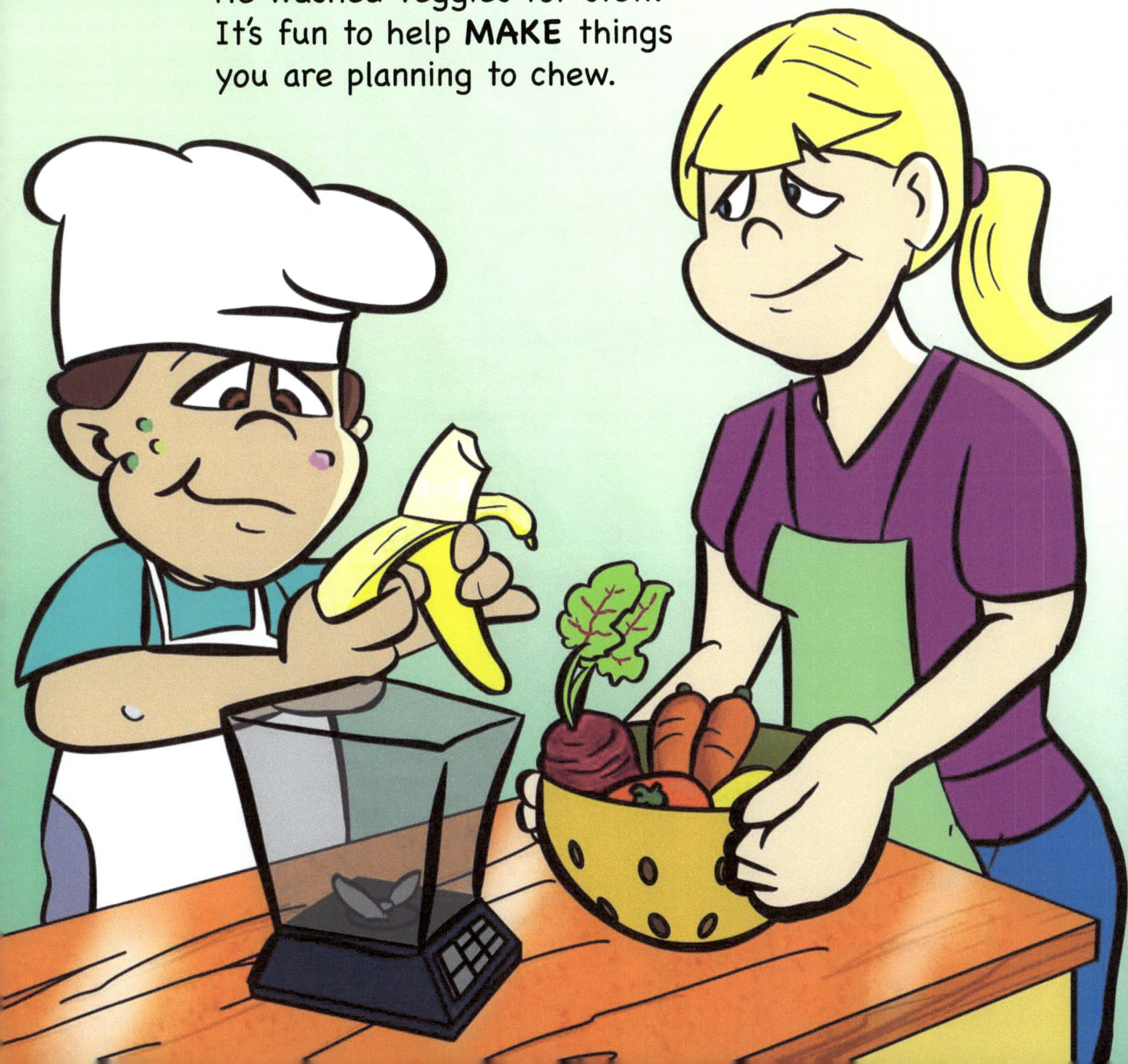

"I'll **MIX** my food with things
that I like to taste.
Some cheese or some lemon
will make it taste great!"

"I'm not used to veggies,"
Nicky thought with a frown.
"I'll put them on pizza
to help get them down."

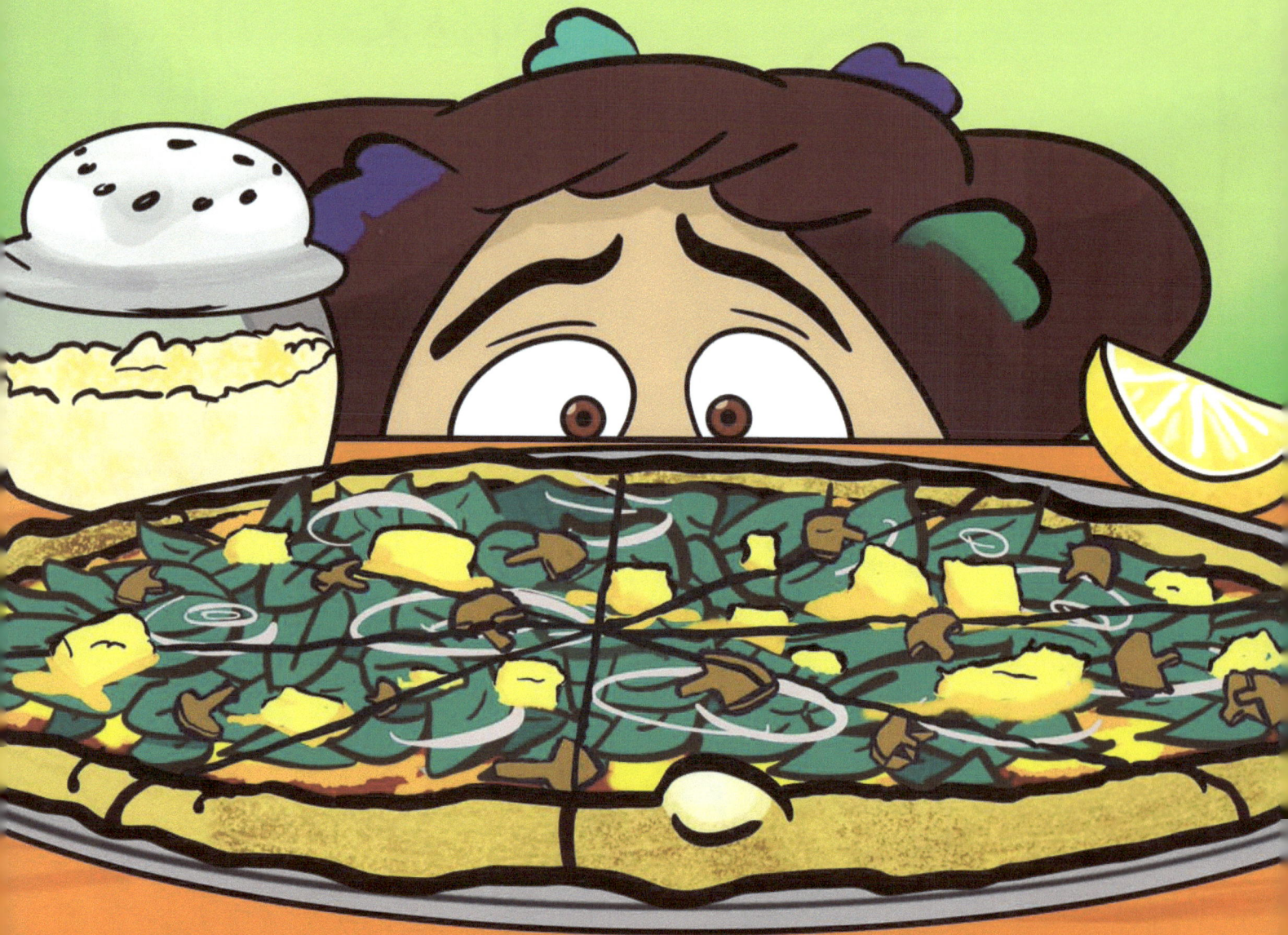

PLAY with your food
to see how it feels.
Build a potato volcano.
Have fun with your meals.

Your carrots can battle
at a ham and cheese castle.
It's a breeze to eat peas
like a scary pterodactyl.

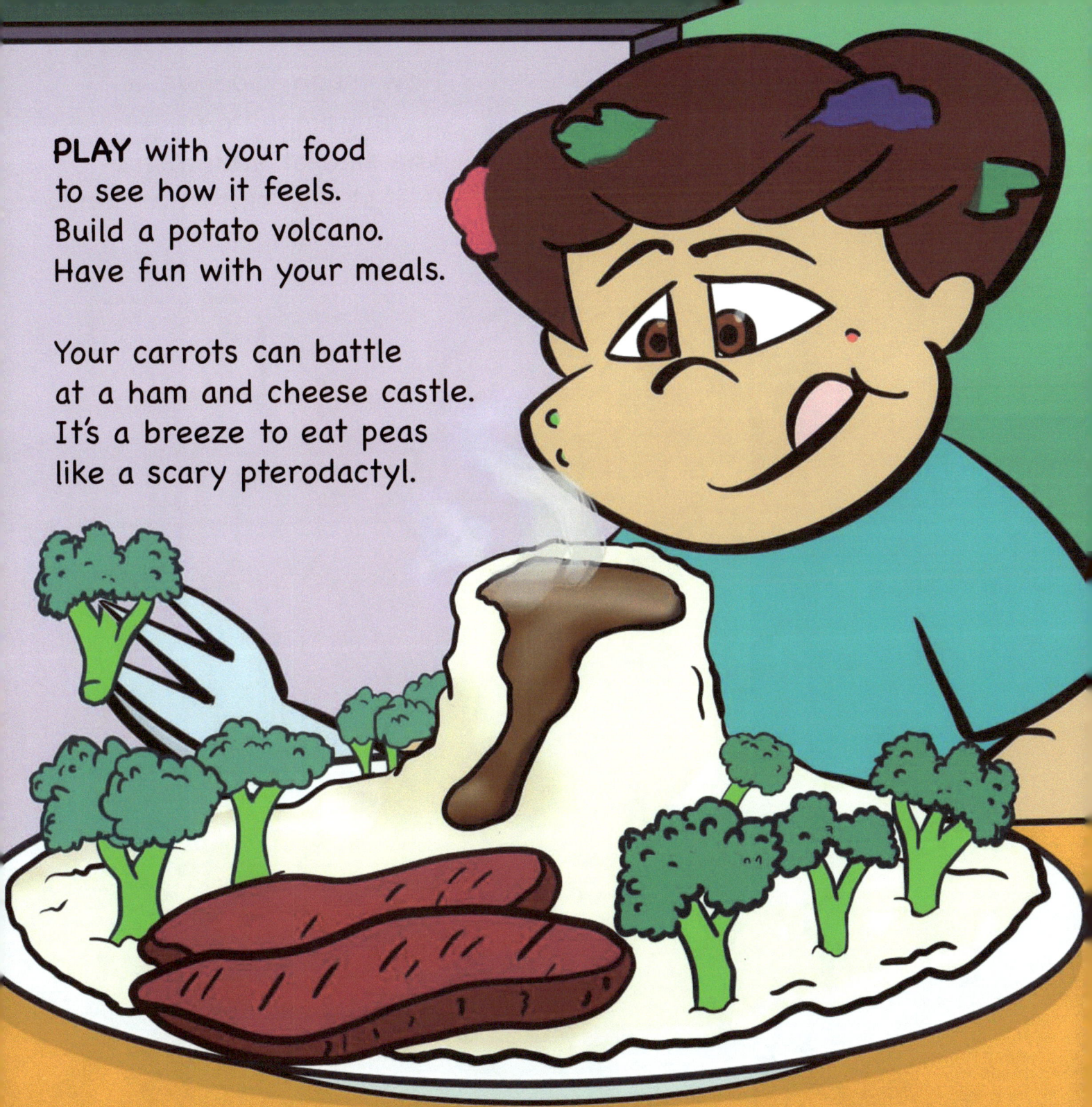

How much food we eat
is very important.
The size of your hand
is just the right portion.

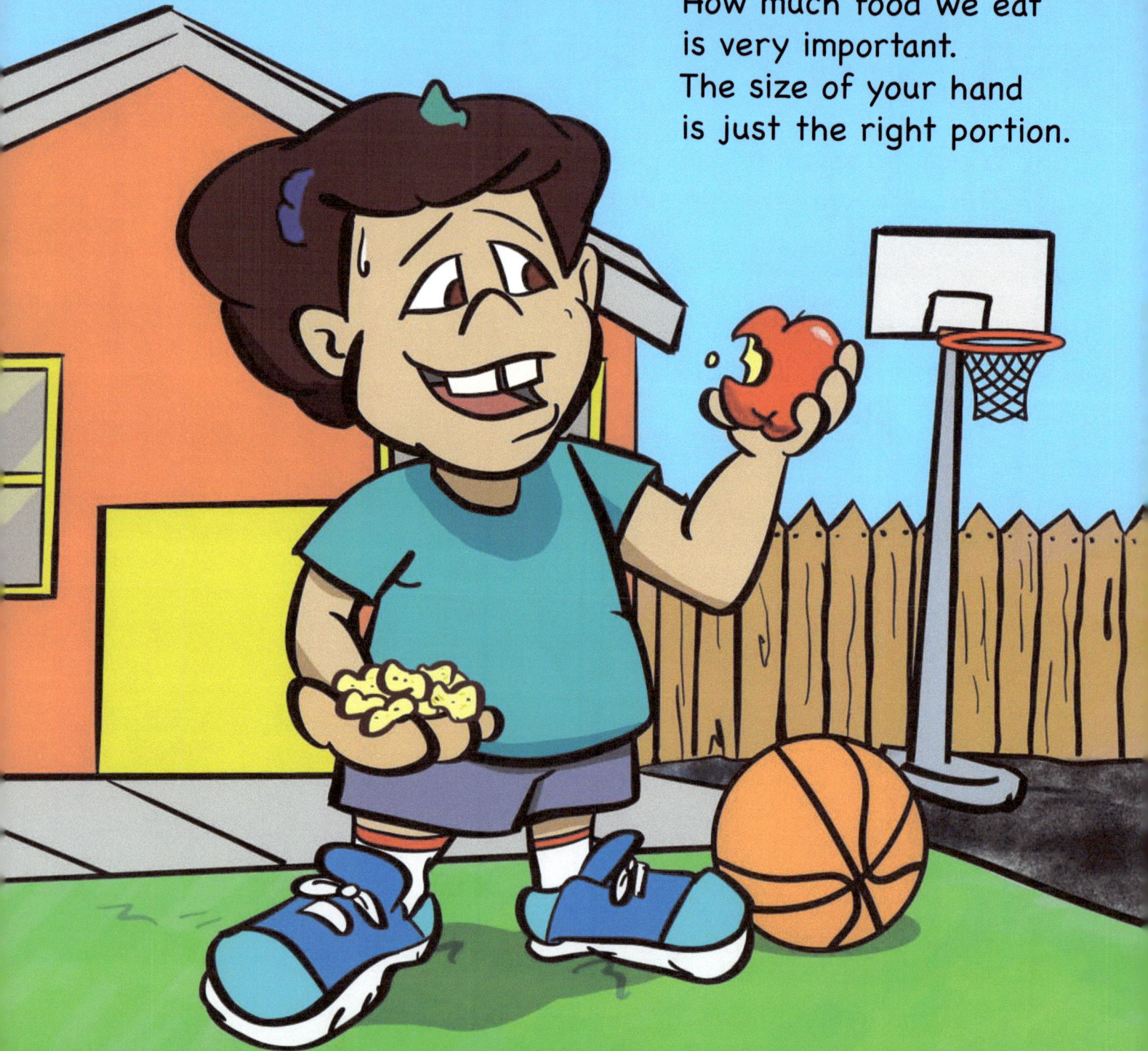

In no time at all
Nicky's hair had changed back.
His skin had cleared up.
He was on the right track.

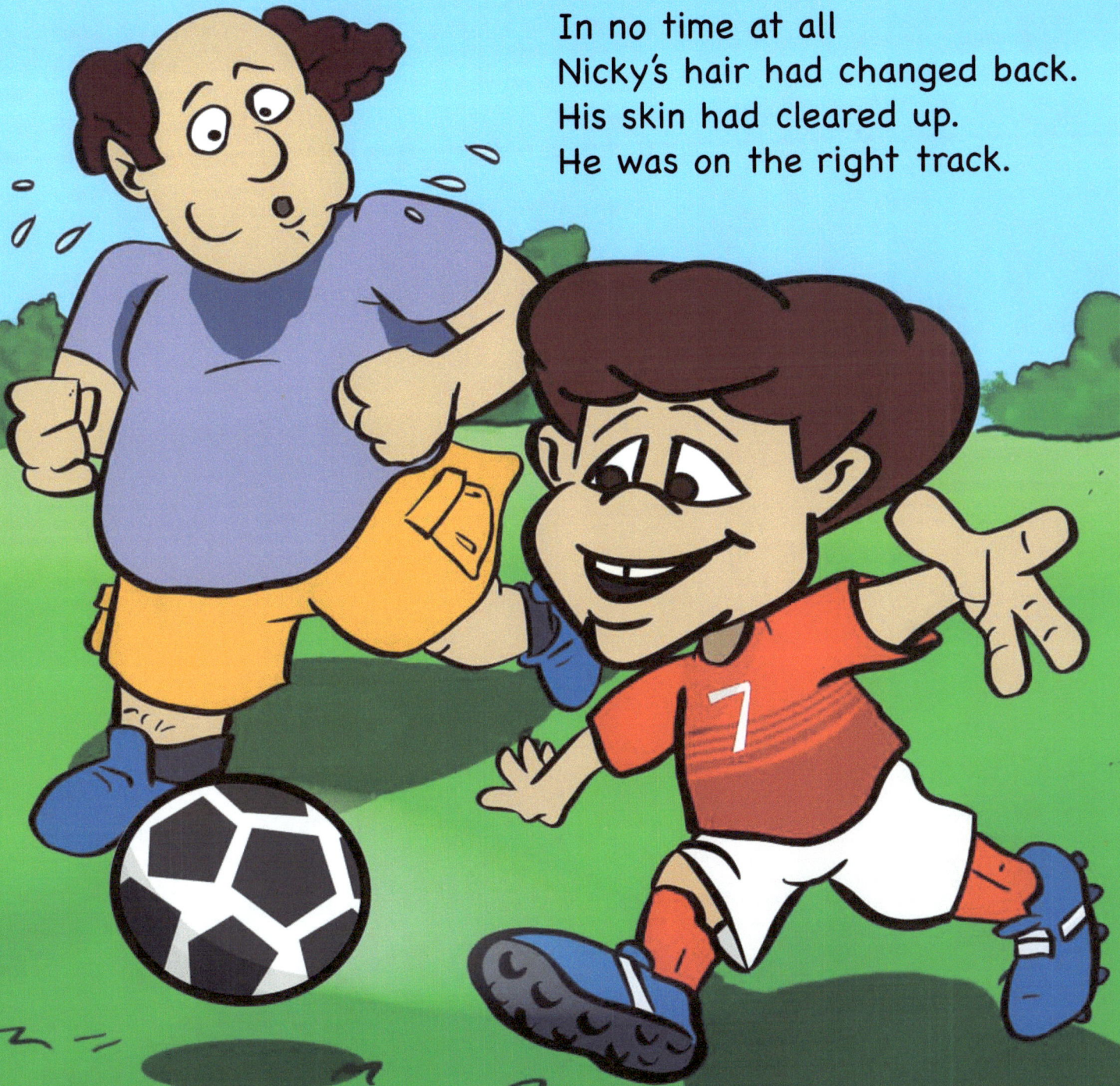

From then on the family ate healthy each day. Mom and Nicky made food that they liked.

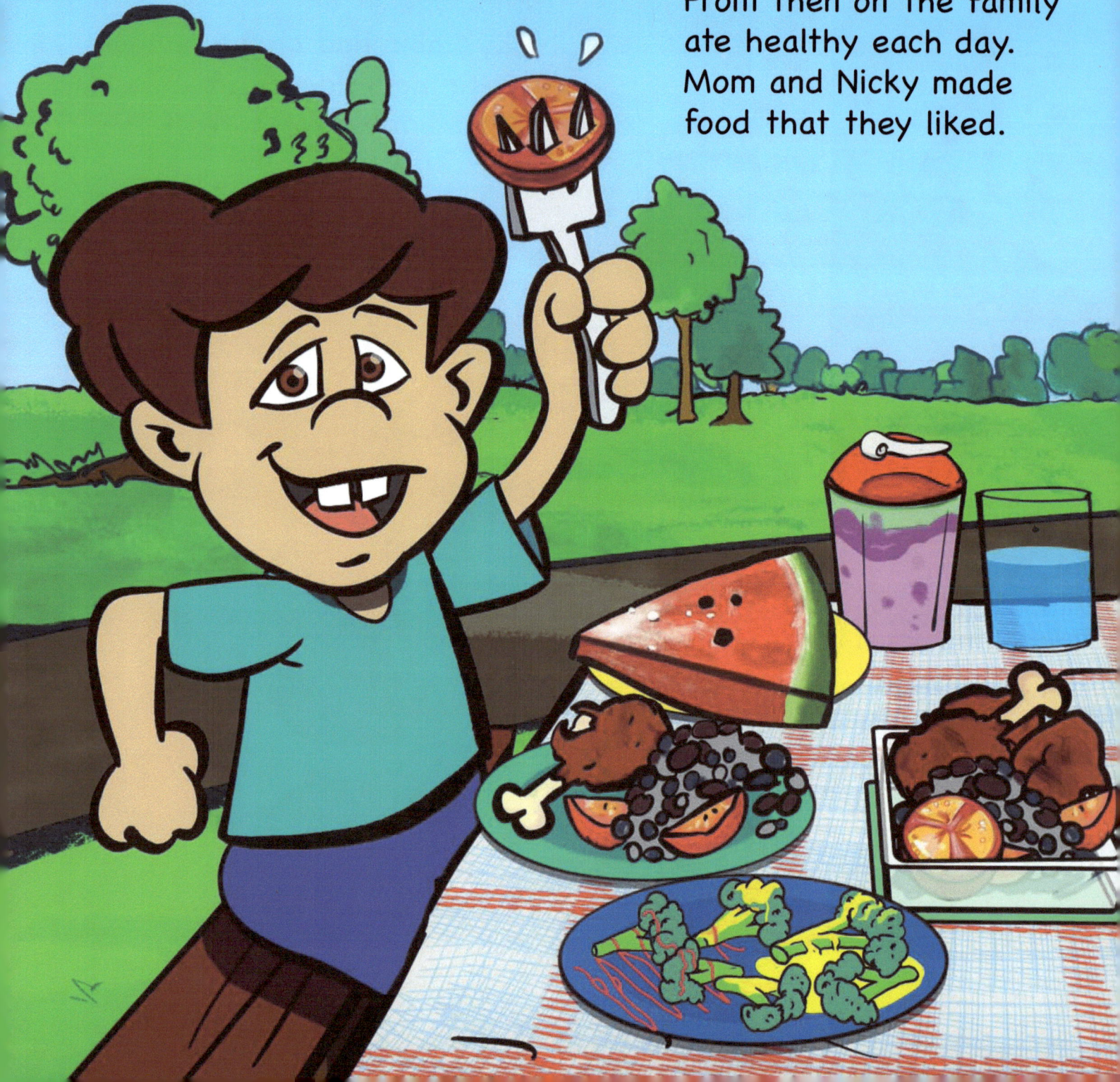

Nicky went outside
instead of online.
He played soccer
and rode
on his bike.

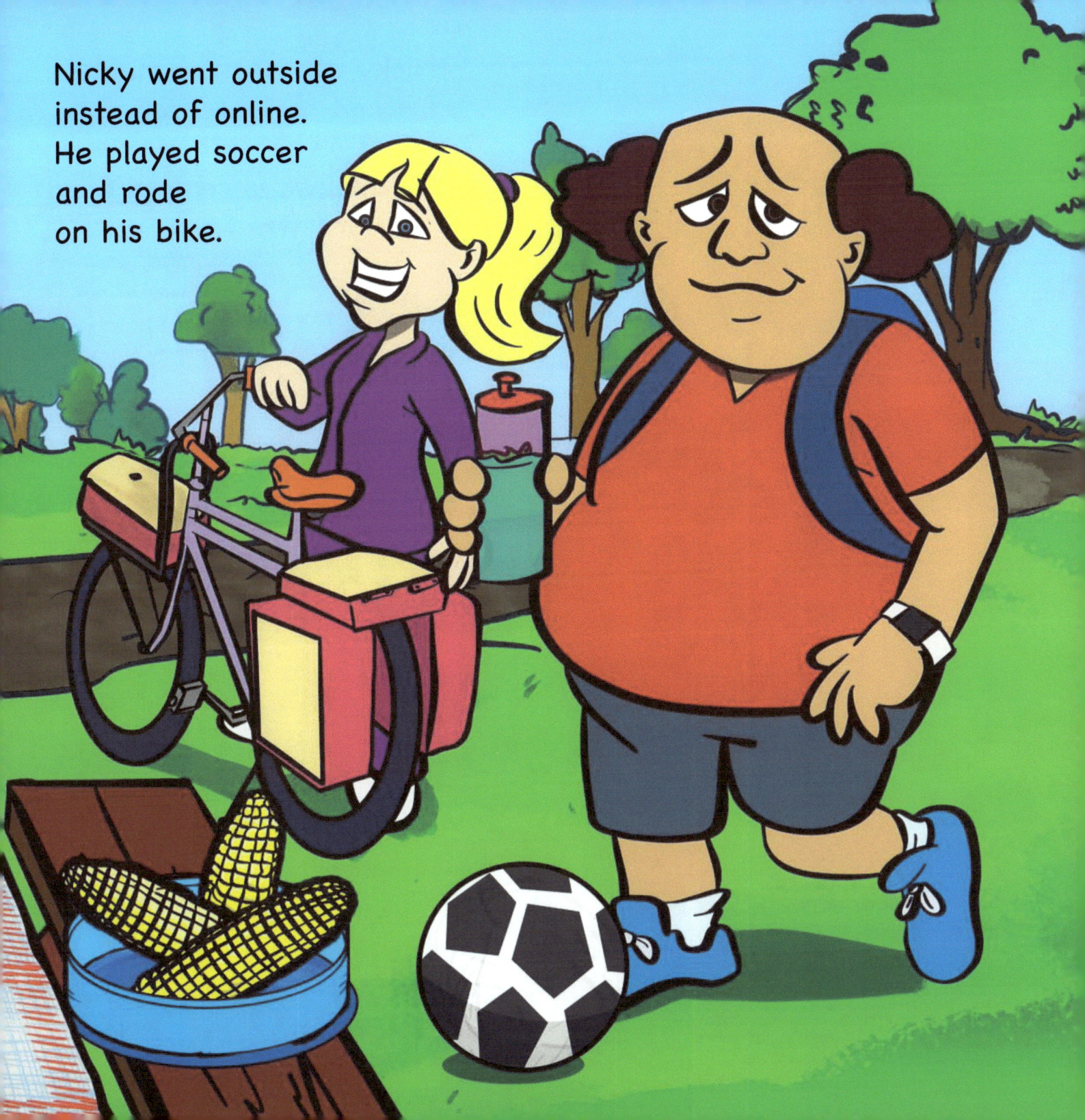

Nicky ate healthy meals
instead of junk food
that's sweet.
Nicky always remembered
"You are what you eat!"

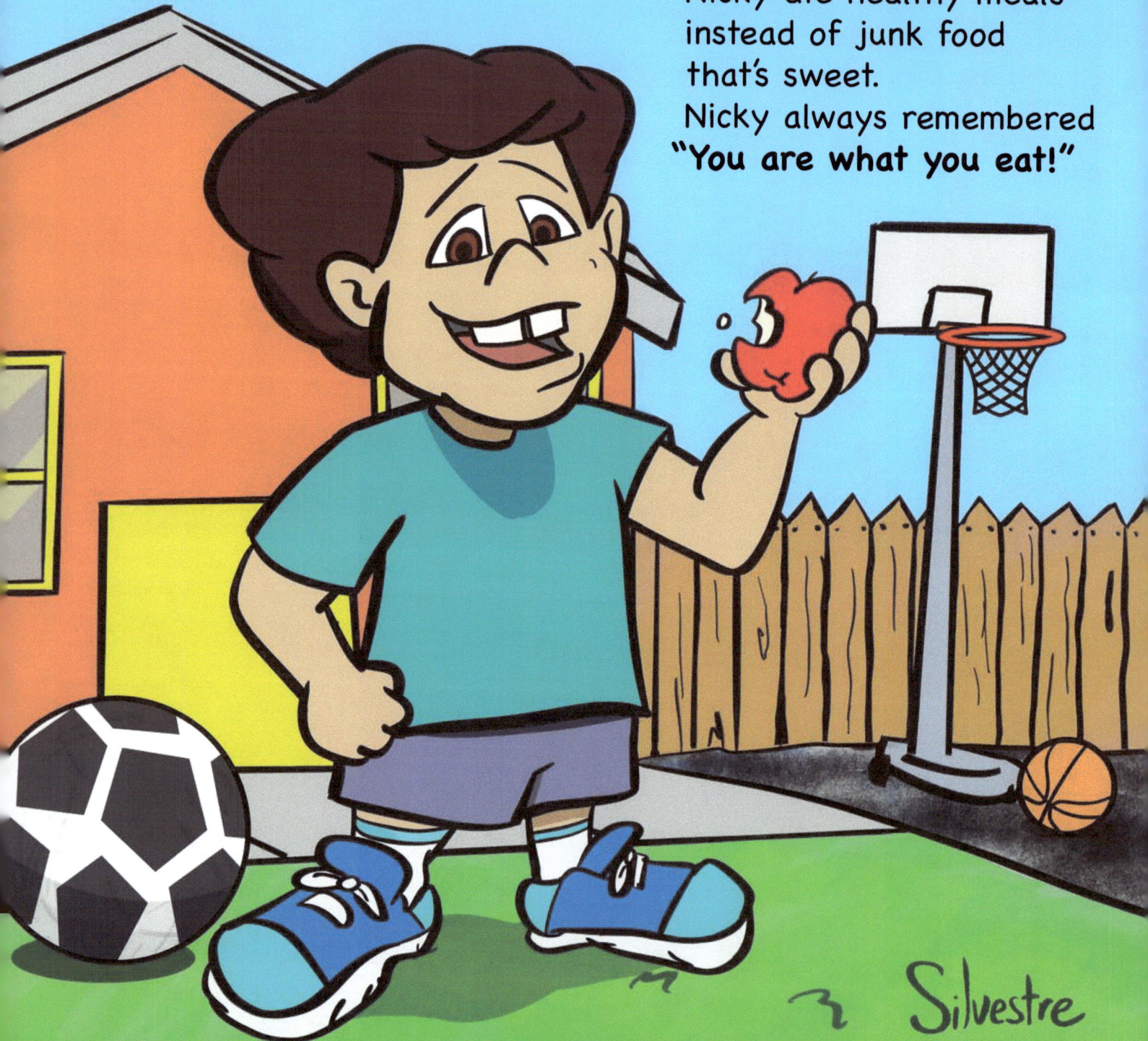

Silvestre

www.ingramcontent.com/pod-product-compliance
Lightning Source LLC
Chambersburg PA
CBHW060857270326
41934CB00003B/177